Occupational
and
Mental Healtn

D1758116

Occupational Therapy and Mental Health

Veena Slaich
Ex-Head
Department of Occupational Therapy
Pandit Deendayal Upadhyaya Institute for the Physically Handicapped
New Delhi, India

Consultant
Occupational Therapy in Private Practice

JAYPEE BROTHERS MEDICAL PUBLISHERS (P) LTD

New Delhi • Panama City • London

Jaypee Brothers Medical Publishers (P) Ltd.

Headquarter

Jaypee Brothers Medical Publishers (P) Ltd
4838/24, Ansari Road, Daryaganj
New Delhi 110 002, India
Phone: +91-11-43574357
Fax: +91-11-43574314
Email: jaypee@jaypeebrothers.com

Overseas Offices

J.P. Medical Ltd.
83 Victoria Street London
SW1H 0HW (UK)
Phone: +44-2031708910
Fax: +02-03-0086180
Email: info@jpmedpub.com

Jaypee-Highlights Medical Publishers Inc.
City of Knowledge, Bld. 237, Clayton
Panama City, Panama
Phone: 507-317-0160
Fax: +50-73-010499
Email: cservice@jphmedical.com

Website: www.jaypeebrothers.com
Website: www.jaypeedigital.com

Publisher: Jitendar P Vij
Publishing Director: Tarun Duneja
Cover Design: Seema Dogra

Occupational Therapy and Mental Health

First Edition: 2012
ISBN 978-93-5025-552-0
Printed in India

Dedicated to

*Millions of psychiatric
cases who get benefited by Occupational Therapy
which is the only remedial process for such
cases that are mentally unwell.
They have been a great source of my inspiration to
write about the role of Occupational Therapy
in the area of mental health to integrate such
patients in mainstream of the nation building with
rest of the society under present day, stresses of
the normal life.*

Preface

Occupational Therapy has been a scientific tool in alleviating the sickness and thereby temporary and permanent disabilities in sufferings of the disabled.

Mental health is a very crucial and important area of human fitness to keep the physical state of the person in order to accomplish tasks in the manner thought and desired by any human being.

Whenever there is any slight or more afflictions of mental capacities, the individual ceases to be called a normal being. There are many exogenous and endogenous causes which give rise to different types of mental ailments like psychotic and neurotic in nature.

The book is an outcome of the class lectures and modified with regard to the final year of Bachelor of Occupational Therapy (BOT) course of four and a half years at Pandit Deendayal Upadhyaya Institute for the Physically Handicapped (PDUIPH), New Delhi, India.

It was always felt that syllabus topics were scattered in different books of psychiatry and occupational therapy and faculty members and students had to waste a lot of time and energy to prepare lectures.

Therefore, it was thought to consolidate the total syllabus in one book as far as possible for the subject of *Occupational Therapy and Mental Health*. While doing so, it can also serve as a textbook on this subject.

Another highlight of the book is the addition of the All India Occupational Therapy Association (AIOTA) conference papers presented over the span of about forty years.

This is, in my view, a first such publication on the said subject in the field of Mental Health and Occupational Therapy in India.

I very earnestly hope that the book will find substantial number of readers, referrals and recommendations as a textbook in various OT schools and their libraries along with libraries of medical colleges as well.

Veena Slaich

Acknowledgments

I acknowledge my sincere thanks to Miss Nisha, a student of MCA, who typed script of this book and my students whose inquisitive queries made the script simple and lucid for easy understanding of the contents of the book.

My heartfelt thanks to my mother who gave me support through day and night along with motivation to pen down my ideas on the subject.

Contents

CHAPTER 1

History of Occupational Therapy in Mental Health

The history of occupational therapy (OT) had it's origin in the 1700's during Europe's "Age of Enlightenment." At this time, radical new were emerging for the infirm and mentally ill. Normally, they were excluded from work activities and were treated like criminals and in local prisons. During this new era concern was given to their mental well-being. This dramatic change can be attributed to two very different men Phillipe Pinel, a French Physician, scholar and natural philosopher and William Tuke, an English Quaker.

Phillipe Pinel was of the belief that morally treating the mentally ill meant treating their emotions. The doctrine of Moral Treatment utilizes occupation; man's goal directed use of time, interests, energy, and attention; in combination with purposeful daily activity for treatment and various forms of literature, physical exercise and work were used as a method to release the mind from emotional stress and thereby improve the individual's activities of daily living.

William Tuke and his family were also redefining the direction of dimental health care. Because Tuke was appalled at the inhumane treatment and the deplorable conditions which existed in the public insane asylums, he developed several principles for the moral treatment of this population. The main approach use was that of the moral concepts of kindness and consideration. He also encompassed the concept of religion which created an atmosphere of family life. Occupations and purposeful activities were prescribed in order to minimize the patient's disorder.

The progression of moral treatment continued into the 1900's as Sir William Ellis and his wife came to be in charge of England's country asylums. This community became a family atmosphere and the men and women both were encouraged to enhance their previous trades to establish new ones in order to support purposeful activity.

Sir and Lady Ellis were able to prove that the mentally ill were not dangerous tools, and were far less dangerous than other unoccupied individuals. The Ellis were also responsible for developing the idea of an after house, very similar to the halfway houses of today. These places functioned as stopping-stones from total care to limited assistance living.

The progressive Era of the Twentieth century in the United States initially was not progressive at all for the mental health field. The moral treatment philosophy had waned during the civil war and nearly disappeared with no one to carry on the philosophy. A lack of concern around of moral treatment was ushered in with the use of sterilization of the "Mental Defectives," the institutionalized insane. Fortunately, in the era 1900s, Susan Tracy, a nurse, employed occupation for mentally ill patients. She also initiated activity instruction to student nurses and coined the term "Occupational Nurse" for this speciality.

Other professionals involved in the rebirth of OT include Eleanor Slagle, a partially trained social worker; George Edward Barton, a disabled architect; Adolph Meyer, a psychiatrist; and William Dunton, a psychiatrist. These professionals, along with Susan Tracy, formed the basics of modern occupational therapy and ensured acceptance as a medical entity with the establishment of the National Society for the promotion of occupational therapy leading to the present day American Occupational Therapy Association.

Occupational Therapy has continued to develop from a deeply-rooted belief in the critical importance of "doing;" of active enjoyment in purposeful activity as a catalyst in the development of self, fulfillment in social membership, social efficacy and self-actualization.

CHAPTER 2

General Orientation and Definition

Psychiatric Occupational Therapy :	The patient is encouraged to develop the attitudes and aptitude which enables him to live as full, useful and satisfying life as possible.
Competent Member of Society :	Should be outside hospital or in community.
Consideration of :	P/H of illness and present illness in relation to his/her personality, intelligence, social and economic background.
Assessment Means :	Should be scientific and should be valuable because patients are people with basic needs of security, adventure, recognition, and response.
Occupational Therapy Help Create :	As normal environment as possible in occupational therapy, patients will not take refuge in over-sheltered conditions. Help patient to meet demands of life outside hospital.

- Frame work for treatment
- The social aspects of mental illness
- Clinical details of mental illness, are necessary for effective treatment in varying degrees.

Rehabilitation Team	: Liaison in staff in psychiatric hospital as good as in General hospital because patient, is less able to develop interpersonal relation for himself.
Occupational Therapy Work with Patient	: To plan and carrying-out treatment as interpersonal relationship
	: With other specialists and team members

- Doctors
- Psychologists
- Nurses
- Occupational Therapist (OT)
- Hospital staff
- DRO (Disablement Resettlement Officer)
- EO (Employment Officer)
- GPs
- SWs
- HWs
- Industrial Managers
- Educational Authorities
- Voluntary Organization
- Relatives of patient. Therapeutic community concept is widened and work is in that framework.

CHAPTER 3

Orientation to Psychiatric Occupational Therapy

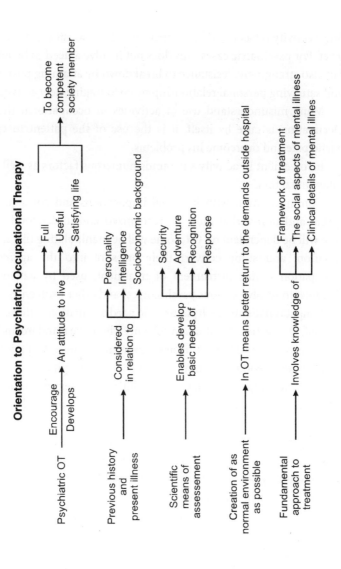

Orientation to Psychiatric Occupational Therapy

Psychiatric OT →Encourage / Develops→ An attitude to live → Full / Useful / Satisfying life → To become competent society member

Previous history and present illness → Considered in relation to → Personality / Intelligence / Socioeconomic background

Scientific means of assessement → Enables develop basic needs of → Security / Adventure / Recognition / Response

Creation of as normal environment as possible → In OT means better return to the demands outside hospital

Fundamental approach to treatment → Involves knowledge of → Framework of treatment / The social aspects of mental illness / Clinical details of mental illnes

CHAPTER 4

Prescription of Occupational Therapy

Since activity is basic to life, occupations release tensions, anxiety and grief. For psychiatric cases, this does not involve a need to be normal but also strengthens resistance to breakdown by attaining purposeful and satisfying personal relationship by encouraging new activites.

Many misunderstand use of activities in occupational therapy. Occupation is cure by itself, it is the use of the patient to enable participate and overcome his problems.

Involvement in activity surrounds numerous factors as well as its inherent factors.

Communication with its social implications and consequences, verbal and non-verbal must be recognized and understood. Some case will be dependent on OT, some will be manipulating therapeutic situation, and some convert their pressure into the aggression. Occupation is just instrument of treatment, used by patient and therapist to resolve various psychological and other problems.

Long stay patients reach platue—So need occupation as therapeutic in itself. Domestic rehabilitation scheme, where the standard and skill in organization and budgeting are important because the patient has to return to freedom in community outside the hospital.

Activities improve social relationships for observation, or as an aid to diagnosis. Many activities achieve more than one end.

Activities are prescribed as under:

a. Activities relating to work: Either to work outside hospital, or training for different job, or for sheltered work in hospital or the community. Work is an essential part of life which provides status and ability to earn livelihood.

b. Work situation:
   - Helps evaluation of physical capacity
   - Manual and intellectual skills
   - Persistence and realiability.
c. Level of motivations: Level of motivation can be understood from building pressures on work and its tolerance.
d. Work worthwhile and essential.
e. Attitude to supervision: Must be observed.

CHAPTER 5
General and Specific Objectives of Occupational Therapist

1. The aims and objectives should be discussed in team of the psychiatric case.
2. Define broad aims of treatment for each patient separately (need based planning).
3. Patient's rehabilitation for return to home/work, or to higher job is to be planned.
4. More immediate aims may be defined which may change from week to week.
5. Design specific activities to evoke particular responses at early stages of treatment.
6. Aims of treatment will depend upon type of cases being handled by the OT like drug addicts, psychopath, epileptics, etc.
7. Plan graded schemes for long stay and treatment cases.
8. Plan programs of psychiatric cases in relation to other profession if need arises as technician and industrialists, occupational therapy teachers, volunteers who help the occupational therapist.

CHAPTER 6

Functions of Occupational Therapy

1. To act in accordance with frame work planned for the treatment of the psychiatric cases.
2. To make the professional standards and judgments in Psychiatric Occupational Therapy by the treating therapist.
3. To have more involvement in paramedical and multidisciplinary discussions concerning psychiatric care.
4. To make program of occupational therapy care flexible to allow adaptation to particular situations.
5. To become involved in certain structured team discussions local levels and in hospital/community.
6. To be seen as continuing treatment, increasingly community centered, except in cases of special need.
7. To make considerable advance in treatment of any psychiatric care.
8. To plan and organize treatment in occupational therapy for psychiatric hospitals, for actually ill patients, the rehabilitation of the long stay patients and for psychogeriatric cases.

CHAPTER 7

Personality of an Occupational Therapist Dealing with Psychiatric Cases

1. Maximum exposed person to psychiatric cases.
2. Role may not be clear always to the client due to complex problems of the cases.
3. Occupational therapist should be clear about his/her role.
4. Therapist should use 'self' to help client.
5. Occupational therapist is a helper and kind may vary.
6. Occupational therapist may be friendly but not a friend.
7. Occupational therapist should try to avoid –ve or +ve authority figuring of himself.
8. Therapist should break through the problem and develop new set of transactions.
9. Therapist should gain client's trust. It helps in motivating the later.
10. Therapist should develop true trust between him and patient by true and effective trust establishing and must be reinforce
11. Therapist should communicate clearly with the patients through out total process of treatment.
12. Therapist should recognize pain under patient's behavior to make easy change process.
13. Therapist's self-confidence and self-knowledge are critical to development of program for patients.
14. Occupational therapy should exhibit effectiveness in treatment approach.
15. Right occupational therapist is who in treatment even makes mistakes and accepts them and is trusted and believed or receives anger.
16. Therapist should recognize issues when arise.
17. Therapist's frame reference will show the issues are tackled.

18. Therapist's should encourage and reinforce to effect a reduction in specific behavior.
19. Occupational Therapist should use occupational behavior from work and sensory integrative approaches.
20. Relationship between Therapist and patient is very important.
21. Occupational Therapist is able to study childhood to maturity behavior better as has the background of the same.
22. She/He should have mature outlook of himself.
23. She/He should have ability to understand patients reactions from her/his situations based on general behavior.
24. She/He should discard superficial reason for inappropriate behavior.
25. She/He should not regard behavior of the patient, as part of illness or usual reaction.
26. She/He should provide an atmosphere of security, reassurance and consistency.
27. She/He should not expose patients to extra over-anxious situations.
28. She/He should understand and except to ways of the patient.
29. She/He should be in a position of understanding presentation, physical condsitions, intellectual response, learning ability, degree of maturity and control, relationships, overt symptoms and behavior, effectiveness of other treatments.

CHAPTER 8

Occupational Therapy Department for Psychiatric Unit

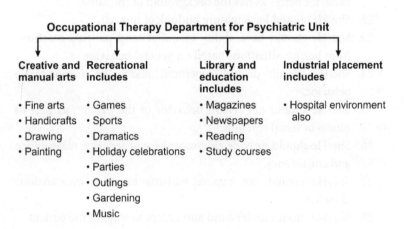

Occupational Therapy Department for Psychiatric Unit

Creative and manual arts

- Fine arts
- Handicrafts
- Drawing
- Painting

Recreational includes

- Games
- Sports
- Dramatics
- Holiday celebrations
- Parties
- Outings
- Gardening
- Music

Library and education includes

- Magazines
- Newspapers
- Reading
- Study courses

Industrial placement includes

- Hospital environment also

CHAPTER 9

Meaning of Activities

Concepts and practices of occupational therapy in mental illness emphasize—interpersonal relationships.

Literature on psychiatric occupational therapy shows over the years that increased emphasis is on therapeutic relationship or on 'use of self' in treatment.

With this focus of interest one perceives diminution of investment in 'the activity' in occupational therapy i.e. end product of art or craft.

Single factor to consider to constitute is that uniqueness of occupational therapy is use of activities or objects.

Psychiatric occupational therapy is used as psychodynamics of activities and the accompanying relationship, one may see inter-personal relationship.

Interpersonal relationships are influenced by factors (contributing element in bringing about any given result) like patient, therapist, group occupational therapy utilizes as an additional component in the form of an activity or object. Influence or impact of this component on others then comprises of occupational therapy experience.

ACTIVITY ANALYSIS

Helps to understand the basic and fundamental psychodynamic character of any given activity. This serves as a guide to evaluate aspects of activity experience.

Use of activities as Psychotherapeutic measure, requires the phenomenal knowledge of unconscious, of nature, meaning of symbols, and of individual psychodynamics, a sensitivity to the probable impact of each of these on one another enabling finally to be able to integrate such awareness into a therapeutic experience for a patient.

The outline below (of activities) helps learner for purposes of assisting them in arriving at basic concepts of characteristics of an activity.

Therefore, broad outline of activity analysis is:

1. Motions:
   - Passive
   - Aggressive
   - Destructive
   - Rhythm, and
   - Size.

2. Procedures:
   - Motor and mental coordination
   - Extent of technical knowledge required
   - Is manual dexterity required or possible?
   - Is there mechanical repetition of procedures? Extent, few or multiple processes required?
   - What is the frequency required for new learning within the procedure?
   - Are there delays or postponement in the process?
   - Must or/can the completion be delayed and/or prolonged? To what extent?

3. Material and Equipment:
   - Resistiveness
   - Pliability
   - Controllability.

4. Creativity and Originality:
   - Extent of expressing feelings
   - Extent of dependence of performance/doing on internal stimuli, creative thinking, planning and implementation
   - Nature or characteristics of opportunity for invention, alteration, original planning and action
   - Nature and extent of external limits/controls to what extent the nature of equipment or material provide structure? To what extent this structure inhibit or control creativity?

5. Symbols:
   - Symbols inherent in the method of procedure, material, equipment, end products
   - What unconscious feelings, needs, drives may be represented by or symbolized in tools, equipments, motions, actions, etc.
   - What is potential of association of hostility and aggression
   - Nature/extent of hostile or aggressive expression on individual directly and symbolically
   - What characteristics of motions, actions, procedures, materials and equipments provide opportunity for hostile or aggressive expression directly symbolically
   - What are the processes for sublimation?
6. Destructiveness:
   - Nature and extent of processes/actions that destroy
   - Is such destruction controlled? What is the nature and extent of this control
   - What tools, equipments, actions etc. may be considered symbolic of destructions, to what extent, what is the nature of this destruction?

CHAPTER 10

Activity Analysis

Activity Analysis

Should provide opportunity for an extent of	Should provide opportunity for constructive expression through the project	Should develop interpersonal relationships	Adaptability or variability in	Contraindication

• Expression of effect and attitude
• Creativeness and originality
	• Hostility
	• Aggression
	• Obsessive compulsive features
	• Expansiveness
	• Narcission
	• Dependence
	• Masculine and feminine identification
	• Regression features
		• With therapist
		• Amount of contract or guidance leading to
		• Amount of Independent performance
		• With the group opportunities for or necessary for working alone
		↓
		Opportunity of working with number of persons <10, opportunity, for exstensive socialization
			• Motion
			• Material and equipment
			a. Resistiveness
			b. Pliability
			c. Controllability
			d. Color-variety
			e. Project:
			  i. Design
			  ii. Number
			f. Chronological levels	

CHAPTER 11

Habit Training in Occupational Therapy

Based on laws of exercise, frequency and recency.

INDICATION

Cannot be started with deteriorating patients, except cooperative with nursing, medical and technical staff and should consult psychologist for ratings. Day should be full and should have routine everyday.

Habit training is an attempt to restore and or maintain those acquired behavior patterns which enable us to perform many tasks efficiently and with little or no conscious thought. In the psychiatric patient, the breakdown of habits frequently accompanies severe intellectual deficit, when the patient is less concerned with his personal life needs, is no longer really interested in his environment or is emotionally unable to feel the effect of his behavior on others.

No OTs can inaugurate a habit training programme for deteriorating patients except in cooperation with medical, nursing and technical staff, and should consult the psychologist about possible ratings to be made in the department or with classes in their charge.

The patient's day must be so organized that it is filled, and it must follow the same basic routine everyday.

Nevertheless, care must be taken that the routine is not so exact in inessentials that patients become rigid unadaptable. Habit training program will be fundamentally similar because the methods are related to basic physiological needs, but may vary in details for one unit to another.

They involve small groups of patients with, usually, one member of staff incharge of varying numbers of patients, but it is not to be emphasized that the ratio of patients to staff must be kept small, to ensure adequate treatment of individual patients.

Care of appearance, as well as bowel and bladder training are impossible. The patient may have to be retaught table manners and normal social customs as well as being retrained to occupy himself. Such aims cannot be realized unless they are willing to be patient and persevering and the training is made easy and pleasant for the patient.

Pleasing appearance should be complimented upon and rewards given progress. These should relate to the patient training and needs, e.g. a personal lipstick, a trip to the canteen, a ward tea-party and they should be given as often as reasonable. Equally, failure should be met with explanation and guidance if necessary, deprivation of privilege. This should not be punitive but used to teach "cause and effect." There should be little time lag between the act and its reward or punishment, but no patient should ever be criticized in front of others, although reasonable criticism by the other patients may be therapeutic.

It must also be remembered that habits can be lost because they are not easy to maintain. The patient should, therefore, has easy access to lavatories, mirrors, brushes, combes and make-ups.

Habit training can be combined with the 'total push' method of treatment which is the continual active encouragement of a patient to participate and cooperate in a group, necessitating a planned and supervised program to cover every hour of the day. The aim is to develop social awareness and responsibility, sense of being an integral part of a group. It involves the re-education of regressed patients and with others, it aims at the establishment of good work habit, development of skills and manual dexterity, and the building of resistance to fatigue. This helps in the exploration of pre-vocational possibilities or, in other cases of long term hospitalization, in assessment for placement in one of the hospital utility department or industrial scheme.

CHAPTER 12

Color Therapy in Psychiatric Interpretations

Different colors have different meanings for normal and a psychiatric patient. The use of such colors by mentally sick persons depicts their inner feelings which are unsaid. So the colors become tools of diagnosing their minds activities/feelings. It is said that:

- Red: Expresses light or mild warm feelings and if thick red is used then it indicates anger
- Blue: When used in less quantity it describes sincerity, masculine feelings, security when used in dark color, it shows sadistic tendencies
- Green: It shows highly creative sense and high emotional development
- Blue and Green: Use of excessive blue shows the masculine feelings and reflects sexuality
- Red and Yellow: Females show good social variety to accept man and flirt more. Males value females
- Black: Depressed/Intellectuals
- Brown: Shows negative aspect of living and is not used by obsessive
- Purple: Shows sincerity and deep depression and experimenting and experiencing with males with good leadership
- Orange: Sacrifice
- Mud Color: It mixes all colors, shows destructive feelings, remote and irresponsible and inadvertently use this color.

CHAPTER 13 — Industrial Therapy to Psychiatric Cases in Occupational Therapy

Therapy through industrial persuits is called industrial therapy (IT).

TYPES

It is of two types:
- Training for open employment
- Training for sheltered employment.

Purpose of industrial therapy:
- Rehabilitation of medium and long-term patients
- Short-term patients seldom need but for the assessment only:
  - To encourage development of work habits
  - To help retention or increase of speed and capacity for work
  - To introduce new skills to those who cannot return to former work.
- Maintenance of work habits in long-term patients:
  - To encourage a normal 'Daily life' pattern for the patients
  - To encourage degree of communication and reciprocity and formation of relationships
  - To offer an opportunity of gaining an appropriate record/ payment and consequent satisfaction
- Suitability of industrial work: This is very important for psychiatric cases if used with discretion:
  - Some patients are put together and some separated for dinning and recreational activites
  - Industrial work given actual live situation work experience.

Such work is useful for schizophrenics, alcoholics, epileptics and psychopaths.

Evaluation: It enables the therapist in assessment of the cases in different settings and actual working conditions in which patient had been before.

Staffing: As under.

Chart

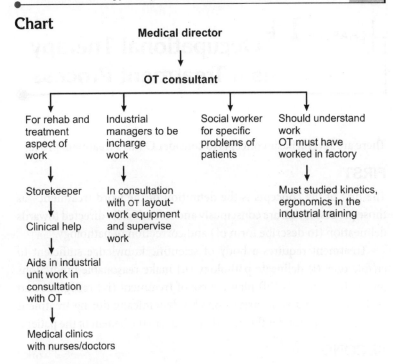

Medical director

↓

OT consultant

| For rehab and treatment aspect of work | Industrial managers to be incharge work | Social worker for specific problems of patients | Should understand work OT must have worked in factory |

Storekeeper
↓
Clinical help
↓
Aids in industrial unit work in consultation with OT
↓
Medical clinics with nurses/doctors

In consultation with OT layout-work equipment and supervise work

Must studied kinetics, ergonomics in the industrial training

Criteria based on:

- Are there enough patients?
- Will workshop fill need?
- Can they be equipped on—Business basis?
- Is transport near—Public/Social
- What is our work in area, have own production line?

Obtaining work

Costing payments

Planning/organization industrial unit

Storage

Payments to workers

Accessibility

Loading/lifting

Transport

Job layout: Correct sequence of whole operation

Quantity and quality control.

CHAPTER 14 Occupational Therapy as a Treatment Process

There are several basic concepts to consider OT as a treatment process.

FIRST

The first of the concepts is the definition of the word treatment—as those processes that are consciously and scientifically directed towards delineation (to describe form of) and correction of pathology.

Treatment requires a body of scientific knowledge sufficient to enable one: (i) delineate pathology (ii) make reasonable predictions on the basic of this (iii) plan course of treatment (iv) recognize and understand what is occurring psycho dynamically during treatment (v) be able to use and influence what occurs to the benefit of the patient.

SECOND

OT as treatment is the concept of the phenomenon of the unconscious. As recognition and understanding of unconscious are fundamental to psychiatry, so are to OT. One-to-one and group relationships affect activities in treatment to the extent that one can understand the impact of unconscious.

THIRD

OT is unique in the use of psycho dynamics of the activities. Use of symbolic and real object relationships and activities mark major contribution of OT in treatment and makes it different from interview and psychotherapy. It is a therapeutic process which relies upon significance of non-verbal communication on psychodynamics of activities, acts as catalyst for development of relationship and intrapsychic experiences to alter and eliminate pathology.

Treatment is changing and ever-dynamic process. As particular needs and problems are worked through, various aspects of the OT experience will assume varying degrees of importance.

OT basic concepts/characteristics may be comprehended and translated into various theoretic frame works like:

- Providing a means of expressing and uncovering unconscious needs, drives, feelings and deal with them in indicated manner
- Providing a means of gratifying needs either directly or by sublimation
- Strengthening ego-defences by assisting the patient to re-establish previous defence mechanisms in a more constructive manner and to learn new satisfactory defences
- Providing ego-growth through distortion of work opportunities in self-concept and body image and to enhance sense of personal identity and worth
- Providing reality from phantasy and to experience consensual (general agreement) validation (confirmation) and agreement on nature of reality
- Exploring interpersonal relationships through opportunities to enter into one-to-one and group relationship, to explore these, to work through interpersonal distortions and to share and communicate with others on a verbal and nonverbal level
- Consolidating gains through continued experimentation, validation and communication in an environment of thinking, feeling and action. Providing opportunity to test one's developing skills in living.

Traditionally, OT works in groups of patients. Sometimes group is so large that it becomes difficult to become involved in a group. When OT functions as a treatment process, the group size should conform to those other therapy groups. It should give sufficient freedom to individual sessions when this is indicated as well as to establish criteria for selection.

Another matter is collaboration with other staff in communication. Ultimate effectiveness of any worker may certainly be measured by the nature and extent of his communication with others who are involved with the patient.

Therapist, psychologist, psychiatrist, psychotherapist must discuss the treatment plan and inherent problems of each case.

CHAPTER 15

Manic Depressive Psychoses

There are hereditary and constitutional factors in the etiology of the affection disorders. It is also said that strong relationship is between Manic Depressive Psychoses (MDP) and cycloid personality.

MANIA

Manic Reactions Affecting Performance and Personal Relationship

Occupational therapy has hardly any role in acute stage of mania because of extreme distractability. Prescription of occupational therapy is advised only after chemotherapy and electroconvulsive therapy (ECT) management. It may be over active with lack of concentration for few minutes, easily irritated and roused to anger with constant interfering in other activities.

The ideas may be profound with lack of idealism. But put more effort into simple job. As they are self assertive, argumentative and have desire to dominate, so disrupt the group.

Occupational Therapy Aims

These will depend upon whether attack was isolated or recurrent. Immediate aims are:
- Reduce activity
- Improve concentration
- Direct dominating tendencies constructing
- Improve social sense
- Prepare him for his previous job and his place in the community with assessment and to select activities for his vocational placement with less responsibility

- As intellect and personality are well preserved, yet employers do not like to employ them due to disruptive previous attacks.

Therapist-patient Relationship

- It is difficult to make relationship with these cases due to lack of insight and desire to dominate. Persuade them to work than directing them
- Self assertiveness should be chanalized constructively, i.e. exploit their talents to the use of hospital and society which offers them prestige
- Avoid opposition directly, handle them firmly with diplomacy
- Accept without involvement argumentativeness as hostility without rancour (bitterness)
- Rapport is strengthened by high work standards and cooperation.

Social Relationships

1. Stress social obligation.
2. Isolation of patients initially till needs to accept criticism.
3. When works with minimum distraction prevent him upsetting others.
4. Choose activity with limited area.
5. On increase of tolerance to criticism, include them in group activities.

Activities

- Tranquillizers and periodic illness has confined patient to hospitals for short time
- Start rehabilitation as soon as patient is ready for it
- Avoid narrow and restive activities to provide composed atmosphere of work
- Short, simple process involvement with rhythmic movements are useful as industrial work, etc.
- Noise, speed, and arguments tend to over stimulate such patients, to avoid fatigue soon

- Uncontrolled and energetic movements do not permit use of heavy and sharp tools
- Give ample of opportunities to gain and restore confidence and adjustment to new work situations.

Contraindications

- Unlimited, uncontrolled movements, i.e. unrestrained dancing, walking, running, crawling, etc.
- Do not switch processes frequently
- Unstrained aggressive outlet like breaking, swimming and demolition work
- Low standard work
- Domination of others.

Liaison (Intercommunication)

- On discharge, patient will need support at day centre or from visits of domiciliary OT in community with concept that readmission is likely.

CHAPTER 16

Obsessive Neuroses

It occurs in rigid and inflexible persons who are not adaptable with extreme sense of orderliness and discipline.

OBSESSIONAL REACTIONS AFFECTING PERFORMANCE AND PERSONAL RELATIONSHIP

The use of ritualistic behavior is handling method designed to retain control over environment and minimise anxiety. There is profound sense of inferiority rituals and counting and repeating actions or phrases, thoughts ruminate and indulge on unprofitable speculations with morbid fears and feelings of guilt. Depression, tension and anxiety are present often as a result of interference of obsessional act. There may be aggressive feelings. These reactions result in:

- Difficulty in starting work, if started their slowness of work to meticulous, perfectionist attitude or repeated checking
- Anxiety when faced by new situations, such as making decisions or thinking creatively
- Difficulty in keeping to time table, although patient is anxious to cooperate
- Distress at being unable to work efficiently, which can result from partial insight into the situation.

OCCUPATIONAL THERAPY AIMS

- Hospitalization for short while
- Fairly deep psychotherapy and protracted (longer lasting)
- Leukotomy in severe cases
- Discharge only after full rehabilitation
- Never full cure of true obsessive case
- As insight develops behavior improves

- Occupational therapy should maintain all useful activity and support to gain improvement by psychotherapy
- Constructive use of perfectionist tendencies
- Occupational therapy may be needed to overcome obsessive tendencies.

THERAPIST-PATIENT RELATIONSHIPS

Unless special role is desired by psychiatrist, she should infuse security, confidence and reduce anxiety. Accept compulsive acts in permissive manner unless menace/danger to others. Patient feels relief after compulsive acts and therapist should use this period to maximum. Impatience increases guilt and failure in patient so the therapist should reduce anxiety. Ritualistic behavior should not be remembered unless done by patient. Occupational therapist should:

- Seek cooperation by discussing full plans
- Be decisive but not authoritarion
- Avoid unpredictable situations and quick decisions by patients
- Give praise and encouragement.

SOCIAL RELATIONSHIPS

Patient should:
- Work with plenty of room where tools and materials are not disturbed but not isolated
- Work with patients who do not disturb the patient
- Encourage general group activities without too much responsibility.

ACTIVITIES

- Activity selection is difficult with varying medical views. Some say repetitive activities have little decision making thus reducing chances of failure and other say that small group activities like play, reading and language study may be advised instead
- Avoid unpredictable situations and indecisiveness or self assertion in relationships with others. Neatness, cleanliness, orderliness high moral standards and high intellect are assets. Support in

group activity can overcome threat of inadequacy. May undertake to menial tasks as long as they are constructive. Like cleaning bathroom daily and washing cups in the deptartment daily. After improvement draw realistic program.

CONTRAINDICATIONS

- Involve continual making of decisions
- Cannot be planned in advance
- Involve surprise.

LIAISON

- Occupational therapist should have full knowledge of other treatments also. Regular reports by occupational therapist for patient must go to doctor. Before and after position of leukotomy case is must to be known. Return to normaly after leukotomy is must to avoid re-appearing of symptoms with constructive activities.

CHAPTER 17

Involutional Melancholia

DEPRESSIVE REACTIONS AFFECTING PERFORMANCE AND PERSONAL RELATIONSHIPS

The disorder is characterized by distortion of physical and mental functions. As described by AJ Lewis, he says 'An adaptation of the organism to an intolerable situation.' The features for occupational therapy consideration are:

- Feelings of inadequacy, gloom, self depreciation and guilt which may amount to delusion of actual crime committed with anxiety and irritability affecting concentration of the concerned
- Physical weakness due to lack of food, interest, insomnia or exercise
- Lack of insight: Patient may deny he is mentally ill with severe hypochondriacal tendencies and complain of bodily ill health not enabling him to work
- Social events and people avoided
- Speech and thoughts affected
- Loss of will power
- Danger of suicide even when improving.

SPECIAL FEATURES IN INVOLUTIONAL MELANCHOLIA

a. Its endogenous depression in men/women at involutional period (involvement) of life
b. Depression in later life increases due to long-life
c. May be an isolated attack which gets cured. May also be considered with cyclothymic depression except when retardation not prominent
d. Regrets at lost opportunities
e. Bizarre and hypochondriacal delusions.

OCCUPATIONAL THERAPY AIMS

- Coordinate Occupational Therapy with ECT
- Treatment is aimed to prevent suicidal attempt
- Distract patient immediately from morbid preoccupations and improve physical condition for resocialization
- Confidence affected if released from hospital without cure of symptoms
- Establish routine as before
- Loss of near and dear one, will cause loneliness or boredome so occupy gainfully
- Prevent institutionalization and dependence on hospital too.

THERAPIST-PATIENT RELATIONSHIPS

- Therapist should not show hostility or rejection towards patient
- Open to view apparent responses lack results into social acceptance and need for satisfaction
- Security may be shown to patient through calm, loving and caring attitude of therapist
- Avoid over attention but give activities which require regular attention
- As depression is cured improve socialization and lessen dependence on the therapist.

SOCIAL RELATIONSHIPS

- Cheerful patients may be clubbed with less cheerful patients
- Hearty, over active or interfering patients may deepen his depression
- Feelings of guilt and unworthiness may be shown on being more communicative
- Give small group responsibility as tolerance improves.

ACTIVITIES

- Interesting activities
- Which are within the capabilities of patient
- Short-term activities

- Externalize feelings with opportunities
- Confined movements with poor posture
- Combine walk with interest, as flower collection for department
- Encourage rhythmic exercises to music and dancing
- Increase socialization on improvement
- Interest in personal appearance, food, nursing care, cooking, etc.
- Suicidal tendencies minimal with improved treatment. Regain confidence in shopping and traveling
- Rehabilitation is aimed at full independence for himself, except for sheltered work in community.

CONTRAINDICATIONS

- Permit to experience failure
- Patient to work in isolation
- Involving speed, noise, confusion of method
- Involving use of unfamiliar, and large apparatus
- Involving use of unsupervised large tools.

LIAISON

- Hospital Treatment with team cooperation
- Allow patient to encourage club/day center
- Contact community occupational therapy for i and ii.

PRECAUTIONS

- Suicidal attempts, should be avoided
- Let not patient wander in lavatories or side rooms when voilation develops.

CHAPTER 18

Reactive Depression

Depression (low spirits gloominess) is generally on individuals due to excessive stress situations. It may also be defined as precipitating circumstance such as a bereavement, an unhappy love affair, or series of frustrations. It can be also observed in many of the physical illnesses.

REACTIVE DEPRESSION (RD) AFFECTING PERFORMANCE AND PERSONAL RELATIONSHIPS

While planning treatment following factors need to be considered:
- Feelings of great unhappiness and inability to face future
- Insomnia, anorexia with hysterical symptoms sometimes
- Lack of concentration and energy
- Early and excessive fatigue
- Dwelling on endless unhappy thoughts and in severe cases danger of suicide.

OCCUPATIONAL THERAPY AIMS
- Divert mind of patient
- Assess needs to combat future difficulties
- House wife may feel depressed due to dissatisfaction of home affairs
- Inability to feed and look after children due to illness or strain
- Psychiatric social worker may assist patient to improve home living conditions. Occupational therapy helps to improve confidence to deal future situations. Assistance in hair dress up, home management, dress making, home-nursing help a lot in women. For men—dress making, home decorating, handyman's work

and gardening. Improvement done in physical conditions help improve confidence and increasing abilities to cope up with live life situations. While patient re-establishes outside hospital extend support.

THERAPIST-PATIENT RELATIONSHIPS

Therapist should:
- Wherever possible show understanding into insight by allowing patient to talk out anxieties and relate to work in hand
- Directions to patient should be clear which do not require patient to make decision till his condition improves
- Encourage independence by gradual withdrawl of support.

SOCIAL RELATIONSHIPS

As change in milieu is useful patient should:
- Encourage to socialize in group activities for lively interchange of ideas and interests
- Encourage to develop confidence of patient by shouldering responsibility of group.

ACTIVITIES

- Relate activities to problems of the patients
- Enjoyable, expressive and creative activities may have relaxing effect on patients
- Successful creative ability stimulate and promote lasting interest and assurance
- Encourage socialization through clubs/group activities
- Relaxation exercises and graded activities advised
- Occupational therapy should see that patient's interests are created to come out of house with cooperation of voluntary workers of area.

CONTRAINDICATIONS

- Do not give difficult activities because they reinforce patients feelings of failure

- Do not give unrealistic activities to patients
- Suicidal tendency case should not be given activities in isolation.

LIAISON

Occupational therapy to be administered with close liaison with psychiatrist, social worker, welfare officer, and occupational therapist working in community.

CHAPTER 19

Drug Addiction

DEFINITION

State of periodic and/or permanent state of intoxication due to repeated consumption of a drug. Its an over powering desire to consume and continue consuming it. There is increasing dose tendency along with marked psychological and physical dependence on drugs which can be seen on withdrawal of the drug.

Drugs are generally taken by emotionally unstable individuals to overcome day-to-day stresses and worries. Such individuals feel that they are making life more pleasant with intake of such drugs, etc. Thus make life unbearable without them, combining organic and functional aspects together. Recently it has come to notice that younger group is more prone to this, as group feeling is quite strong at that age. Those who are addicts they infect others also to join them.

Some centers have been opened near the hospitals so that such cases are taken care of fully and deal patients with psychotherapy. Addicts without work loiter around or stay out of such centers. Occupational therapist here harnesses abilities whatever remain. In patient treatment may become necessary if symptoms demand or the patient accepts withdrawal treatment. Some take heroine and cocaine and a small number amphetamine and barbiturates. Such addicts are from broken homes or other problems with parents. They are antisocial, plausible and selfish and do not cooperate during treatment. Unresolved sexual problems are also a cause sometimes. Before admission to hospitals results, in many addicts, who loose careers and jobs like this.

AIMS OF OCCUPATIONAL THERAPY

- Withdrawal of drug
- Physical rehabilitation, includes improvement in physical condition
- Occupational therapy should distract attention from discomfort psychologically and physically and should support patient
- Encourage good work, habits and pleasure in life
- Arrange employment after discharge.

THERAPIST-PATIENT RELATIONSHIP

Addicts are inadequates, little tolerant and frustrated from life.

CHAPTER 20

Alcoholism

Prolonged use of alcohol (toxin) results in acute or chronic psychoses. This kind of a person is compulsive drinker who seeks treatment before his condition has gone bad due to loss of job or family position/conflict. Root cause may be psychopathic condition or neurotic. This need may start due to social pressure or inner need. Some time in persons with strong emotional conflicts can gain it as compulsive dependence. Alcohol is taken by emotionally unstable person.

Inhibitory areas of frontal lobes are compressed by alcohol whereby judgment is lost with false feeling of confidence. Deep emotions anger, resentment and aggression may be openly expressed and he feels relieved of symptoms till he sobers down when remorse (deep sorrow of having done wrong) follows to drink more to reduce tension.

This vicious circle continues which later becomes physiological need to maintain alcohol level to which body has adjusted.

AIMS OF OCCUPATIONAL THERAPY

- Alcohol can be left while in hospital
- This is a long term improvement to be sustained with difficulty
- Intramuscular injection can be used as conditioned reflex which produces emesis (regurgitates stomach contents) or drug as antabuse which destroys taste for alcohol
- Many advocate psychotherapy than resorting to 3 above
- Put alcoholics together to discuss their problem to find out solutions
- Patients may be encouraged to join Alcoholics Anonymous (AA).

Basic occupational therapy aim is to make their return to normal life as soon as possible. Give group activities to make them leave need to drink. After insight develops they can help themselves to resolve inadequacy feelings and do constructive work. If previous job is lost, work on employment opportunities.

THERAPIST-PATIENT RELATIONSHIPS

- Develop therapeutic relationship with alcoholic to overcome feelings of his short coming
- Rationalise his behavior and minimize his problems
- Guilt and depression comes due to suffering caused to others
- Encourage and induce self-respect in patient.

SOCIAL RELATIONSHIPS

- Group work is best though these cases find it difficult and do not participate fully
- Encourage to accept responsibility
- Plan activity groups—socialization, communication of ideas and communication of feelings.

ACTIVITIES

- Individual activities to foster individual interests
- Establish work routine in patient before discharge
- Clerical/industrial/manual work is useful with regular work pattern
- Activities like children's party, providing pot plants for old patients to look after, can be given towards end of the treatment
- Give graded activities to improve general health.

CONTRAINDICATIONS

Activities which:
- Isolate the patient
- Provide means to take alcohol (money, access to methylated spirits, etc.).

LIAISON

- Staff of alcoholics unit must work together
- In good therapeutic relationship patients confide better and tell their problems which they could not express
- Common problems like home situations, financial position of patient's family, etc. and information should be passed to social worker and doctor both.

CHAPTER 21

Hysteria

It is fake symptom production of any kind in any individual—ladies and girls being more in incidence. Common causes are emotional involvement of an attempt disguised, to gain advantage by showing some physical symptoms with incidence of pre-occupation ideas.

HYSTERICAL REACTIONS AFFECTING PERFORMANCE AND PERSONAL RELATIONSHIPS

- Imitation of any physical/psychological symptom—paralysis, anesthesia, memory loss, torticollis, etc. lead to poor concentration
- Anxiety if physical symptoms partly resolve the conflict
- No depth of emotions, i.e. la belle indifference with egocentricity to show high in obligation with others, resulting into lack of responsibility
- Suggestibility high, adaptability over, dependent/attention seeking traits.

AIMS OF OCCUPATIONAL THERAPY

Depends on history of the case and effect of psychotherapy:
- Find alternate means to fulfill psychological needs
- Introduce activities which increase confidence and sense of achievement
- Activities which encourage responsible attitude
- Diminish need for compensation by assisting patient to be more socially acceptable manner
- Provide treatment for established deformities and pre-vocational exploration where residual disability exists.

THERAPIST-PATIENT RELATIONSHIPS

Approach needs skill:

- It is necessary to differentiate between real and fake pain (attention seeking)
- Do not show sympathy
- Withdraw concessions/relaxation in behavior gradually.

In Addition, Occupational Therapist Should

- Evaluate patient's conception of illness
- Gradually minimize importance of physical symptoms
- Be kind, firm, attention giving where necessary
- Praise achievements
- Do not tame possessive tendencies
- Overcome inability to accept explanations and
- Observe patient in various situations.

SOCIAL RELATIONSHIPS

Do not place these patients, in groups where they become center of sympathy and not with similar groups.

- Place in group who can accept any overt hysterical symptoms
- May be encouraged to accept responsibility.

ACTIVITIES

- Assess physical capacities carefully to give graded work/activity. Initially give activities with in their capacities
- Achievements compensate for weaknesses to throw hysterical symptoms
- Ego-centric appeal activities to be given to divert mind to produce symptoms
- Activities like dress making/tailoring, wooden toys making and gardening, etc. should be encouraged
- Activities which involve intellect should be promoted
- Give graded physical effort activities
- As patient improves give responsibility sharing activities

- Give activities which have little show-manship like, selling magazines, etc.
- Arrange realistic work situations
- Prevocational exploration to be undertaken, where necessary.

CONTRAINDICATIONS

- Activities below and beyond patient's capacity
- Activities permitting boredom
- Do not allow patient to gain others approval
- Re-informing any physical disabilities
- Activities which appeal immediately and are temporary escape from planned program.

LIAISON

- Correlate treatment with psychotherapy—Upgrading skill and concentration to progress
- Fatigue/irritability due to psychotherapy increase, boredom.

CHAPTER 22

Anxiety Neuroses

People with over anxiety suffer from this as a result of hereditary or environmental factors.

ANXIETY REACTIONS AFFECTING PERFORMANCE AND PERSONAL RELATIONSHIPS

It is chiefly characterized by feelings of tension, anxiety, fear or specific phobias without any adequate reason.

Symptoms like tremors, loss of muscle tone, rapid breathing, sweating, etc. affect performance. Loss of weight due to poor appetite thus affecting general condition (GC). Patient may collapse in serious condition.

Psychological symptoms—Irritability, insecurity with inferiority feelings seen. Patients are over susceptible and overreact to stress. In occupational therapy these reactions result in:

- Fear of starting any activity project
- Doubt power of achievement
- General lack of interest, slowness, lack of persistence and concentration
- Patients aim high to cover feelings of inferiority
- Lack of energy and initiative because of lack of capacity to turn from unpleasant ideas
- Tries to escape into invalidism to avoid stressful situations.

OCCUPATIONAL THERAPY AIMS

- Assist patient to adjust to hospital life
- Help to regain self confidence, lessening of tension, influencing him into personal and group situations
- Provide energy release to accept/resolve anxieties

- Improve physical conditions
- Assess capabilities of patient to sustain stress/unexpected difficulties
- Gain/sustain patient's interest in selected rehabilitation program and
- Create new interests to carry on after discharge.

THERAPIST-PATIENT RELATIONSHIPS

- Occupational therapist to see patient soon on admission without hurry to start treatment because before patient is ready to accept new situation to avoid serious resistance. Occupational therapist should be prepared to adopt any role as desired by doctor to support his treatment and should establish confidence
- Be friendly but decisive without placing much responsibility on patient
- Avoid provocation of symptoms except with delebration
- Encourage sufficiently to develop self-consciousness to therapeutic relationship
- Psychotherapy increases insight so give opportunity to discuss attitudes to work.

SOCIAL RELATIONSHIPS

- Place patient with small group
- Provide increasing responsibility within group and
- Introduce him to wider social field.

ACTIVITIES

- Avoid too long isolated activities
- Avoid competitive activities unless improved
- Work standard should be estimated within his capacities
- Give less demanding activities
- Give familiar activity first as there is less confidence
- Muscle tension varies—Large movements better than small ones
- Gardening good for absorbing energy
- Games help to release tension
- Relaxation exercises useful if to be continued at home on discharge

- Short duration activities should be given—hair dressing, flower arranging or making a garment
- Make above activities more realistic to gain/develop confidence for leisure groups, activities of daily living (ADL) and social groups.

CONTRAINDICATIONS

- Avoid activities beyond patient's capacity
- Avoid long duration activities
- Avoid isolated activities on any fixed apparatus
- Avoid competitive activities
- Avoide activities which are too tiring as per patient's physical state.

LIAISON

- All staff members should handle patient consistently
- Occupational therapist should know of tension relieving drugs — To speed improvement, to help plan patients progressive rehabilitation.

CHAPTER 23

Psychosomatic Disorders

Two main types of Psychosomatic Disorders are: (i) those in which emotional disturbance causes symptoms and (ii) in which emotional disturbance plays on physical symptoms present already. This wide group covers patients who have developed genuine physical illness as an unconscious method of avoiding anxiety and gaining sympathy and approval or as an escape from difficult problems.

Psychosomatic disorders cover a good range of the symptoms, mainly of asthma, migraine, ulcers, urticaria, neurodermatitis and persistant diorrhoea. So treatment cannot be generalized.

PSYCHOSOMATIC REACTIONS AFFECTING PERFORMANCE AND PERSONAL RELATIONSHIPS

Individuals who are over-anxious, over-conscientious and rarely aggressive. Aggression may be covered as reaction formation as timidity. Fear and anxiety are underlying causes to produce physical symptoms which might have originated in early stage and stress/strain makes them evident clinically.

Occupational therapy should remember that—(i) physical illness is real-pain and fatigue (ii) performance in occupational therapy is affected at two levels—(a) Physical disability and (b) Underlying fear and anxiety.

OCCUPATIONAL THERAPY AIMS

- Due to diversity of there disorders—Understand patient fully
- Main aim is to relenquish patient's defence mechanisms in favor of activities which are not neurotically motivated
- Give constructive work to avoid patients being preoccupied with physical symptoms and lack of confidence

- Give an outlet of aggression—If physical symptoms contribute to asocial or antisocial attitudes, resocialization may be important aim of treatment.

THERAPIST-PATIENT RELATIONSHIPS

By the time patient reaches hospital his symptoms are ingrained. Patient's past experience has been to awake sympathy and attention which is followed by impatience, annoyance and finally rejection. Rejection increases tension and production of symptoms.

Occupational therapy should accept patient with complaints without pity or concern (i) reassurance and (ii) encouragement is the key. As these patients are highly suggestible so no new ideas should be given to avoid physical symptoms. After patients has poured out his complaints—Occupational therapy should try to divert his attention to avoid showing undue interest in his symptoms. Approach patient when he is in less-interested mood, so feels accepted as a person and not as ill phenomenon.

- Give time to understand personality involved
- Be firm and gentle to accept hostility and irritability
- Reward and recognize the accomplishments
- Reassurance and support to be withdrawn gradually as need lessens.

SOCIAL RELATIONSHIPS

- Avoid isolation at all costs
- Introduce early to group activities
- Gradually give responsibilities within group
- Other patients may project difficulties accusing staff of no concern
- Should be dealt with doctors in group meeting.

ACTIVITIES

- Should be within the capacity of patient giving opportunity of self-expression
- Free painting and modeling give outlet to aggression and also gardening wood and metal work

- Activities encouraging cooperation in group–cooking meal, social and recreational activities
- On patient's improvement—Realistic activities should be introduced
- Leisure persuits may be met where patients interact with others in normal medium.

CONTRAINDICATIONS

- Increasing dependence on therapist by prolonging learning new persuits
- Activities that are closely structured and allow no freedom
- Give so much freedom that patient has no basic routine to support him
- Activities aggravating somatic symptoms thereby drawing attention to it
- Activities which are beyond patients capacity.

LIAISON

- Contact with psychiatric social worker (SW) essential to coordinate occupational therapy at home
- There may be problems, when psychosomatic case is placed in physical unit in any group activity
- As soon as patient is in a condition to go to dept, he may be engaged with other patients of rehabilitation group.

CHAPTER 24

Psychopathic Personalities

As per mental health Act United Kingdom (UK) 1959, the criteria for such disorder is social than medical or psychiatric.

Behavior is characterized by: social aggression, there is inability to profit from experience, self-centeredness, poor judgment, emotional responses facile (moving), lack responsibility, aggressive, under pressure, and repeat mistakes often. Immaturity is common in aggressive type.

In many cases such tendencies vanish in late 20's and 30's which suggest that delay in maturation is predisposing factor.

There are two groups of this disorder (i) aggressive (ii) inadequate. Treatment of both have fundamental problems. Inadequate are less dangerous than aggressive type and may have more serious repercussions of their inadequacies.

PSYCHOPATHIC REACTIONS AFFECTING PERFORMANCE AND PERSONAL RELATIONSHIPS

Above symptoms affect OT care of the patient which include:
- Camouflaging failures by apparent competence
- Present is significant and lack planning in life
- Cannot evaluate behavior and himself
- Lack of reliability and perseverance (to continue despite odds).

OCCUPATIONAL THERAPY AIMS

Due to lack of learning from experience—treatment in a permissive environment will be difficult. Group psychotherapy may help. Treat by conditioning based on principle—If no yardstick of ethics exist where by patients can judge his acceptable or unacceptable behavior. Giving/withdrawing privileges must be done.

Occupational therapy should help patient to make aware of his responsibilities and ability to combat antisocial impulsiveness. This helps more for inadequate person than for aggressive, as for later more therapeutic program should be there. Occupational therapy should have considerable control over patient with understanding.

THERAPIST-PATIENT RELATIONSHIP

Such patients gain sympathy of staff and patients as they are plausible (apparently right). With superficial contact, you can plan rehabilitation program for these case. Therapist should grasp control of case with friendly attitude and showing no aggression. Patient should be explained what is expected of him during activity and wilfull deviation by patient should be corrected immediately. Restraint and resentment on authority should be taken calmly by therapist.

SOCIAL RELATIONSHIPS

- They make good first impression
- May be rejected by others on their being argumentative
- Generally psychopaths are above average IQ
- These cases exhibit care and concern for others to gain approval of staff to get privileges granted
- They identify themselves with staff-keep in control to encourage them to work
- Constructive persuits without exploiting others
- Do not give position of authority.

ACTIVITIES

Psychopaths are physically fit persons so full work with community work should be planned. Jobs in the sheltered workshops and depaertmental stores should be provided. Reward good work with recreation and with interesting work. Social clubs will provide exposure for responsibility, e.g. treasurer. Poor work and bad behavior may be immediately demonstrated in responsibilities. Reward must follow quickly. Some psychopaths have skills in creative arts and manual abilities and as in music, engineering or experimenting with new inventions, and provide scope for creative expression.

CONTRAINDICATIONS

- Activities encouraging unrealistic attitude to life
- Allow patient to work in unsupervised situation
- Permit a low standard of work
- Permit the patient to dabble (engage superficially) with job rather than see it through beginning to end
- Allow him to exploit others.

LIAISON

As they are clever manipulators, occupational therapy should work in close liaison with full therapeutic team.

CHAPTER 25

Senile Dementia

It is a psychotic condition resulting in part from cerebral deterioration. Students view it as due to growing age progression and patient fails to the treatment given to mentally normal geriatric case.

Many symptoms are exaggerations of old age, lack of insight due to senility which is a concern of treatment. With normal elderly person—The aim is to encourage purposeful life with high degree of independence. Peace of mind and body are the first consideration while treating any senile person.

Send these patients to department in early condition only. Later treat them in wards only in homogenous groups, as confusion, leading to wandering, incontinence, etc. and lack of normal inhibitions may cause difficulties with other patients.

OCCUPATIONAL THERAPY AIMS

Alleviate anxiety which is natural outcome of confusion. Cap reserve good habits which remain. Maintain physical tone as much as possible because they are frail for exertion.

THERAPIST-PATIENT RELATIONSHIP

Occupational therapist should adapt her approach to the condition and extent of grasp of situation. As patient fails to recognize places/persons, therefore, each treatment session is new for each time before any signs of grasp and recognition are seen in the patient.

SOCIAL RELATIONSHIP

These are impossible to achieve as of disorientation of the patient but group activities may be used where ever possible.

ACTIVITIES

- Give activities like exercise
- Habitual skills may be also successful than the new ones
- Conditions including physical, heart, eyesight and hearing affect choice
- Every step is taught a fresh
- Memorising may cause stress and anxiety.

For women: Needle work, crocheting, knitting, etc. and mending may be practicable, domestic work like, laying table, dusting, washing, etc.

For men: Wood work, industrial work, gardening, etc. may be useful.

- If the complete operation is not possible then single operation may be given—As sanding and sorting raw material Radio, TV, "sing song" can help stimulate patient and turn his attention from narrow confines of ward
- Habit training necessary for each patient to follow their routines to develop security through familiarity
- Occupational therapist should be a vital part of the total program
- Good habits should be encouraged like, easy access to lavatories a must.

Dementia is irreversible and progressive, the patient becomes more unable and more emotionally labile so occupational therapist while helping him to work at highest level see decline of mental and physical condition. Modify activities to avoid stress.

CONTRAINDICATIONS

- Learning new processes
- Judgment and initiative
- Use of dangerous tools, equipments and materials.

LIAISON

Collaborate with ward nursing staff to plan full day of the patient including small ward tasks also. Volunteers may help to develop friendship and bringing in of outside interests.

CHAPTER 26 Role of Occupational Therapy in Rehabilitation of the Mentally Ill

Interest in Mental illness—In last few years drugs have succeeded in their attitude concerning the reversibility of the process of mental Illness and has made more patients available for treatment and rehabilitation.

Rehabilitation concept in psychiatry ranges between vocational placement and training to almost all aspects of treatment planning and programming.

Rehabilitation concerns mainly in developing skills and capacities which may be directly related to successful economic and social functioning in community outside hospital.

Occupational therapy bridges the gap between hospital and community by assisting the patient during treatment sessions.

As occupational therapy is small part of rehabilitation effort, so rehabilitation is one portion of the role and function of occupational therapy.

Rehabilitation is not only impact of psychologic impact of work but is in our culture, it is man's source of preservation and livelihood.

OBJECTIVES OF OCCUPATIONAL THERAPY

- While involving in any rehabilitation program of any patient, it is necessary to study working knowledge of social, cultural and economic structure of the community to which patient will return
- Any worker of this field must know psychological meaning of work in our culture
- To have sufficient knowledge of psychology, psychiatry and sociology to assist others in helping the patient to establish reasonable and meaningful social, vocational and economic goals and to work with the patient—Towards attainment of the goals

- Nature of occupational therapy and understanding of therapist of psychologic significance of action and objects provide a means for evaluation of skills and difficulties in relating to and sharing with peer group and authority
- Evaluation and assessment of patient's integrative capacities, organizational ability, capacity for abstract or concrete thinking, manual dexterity skills is essential
- Success of rehabilitation is dependent on structure and therapeutic philosophy of the institutions
- Most concepts emphasize the necessity for cooperative effort within a milieu conducive to shared goals and concepts, inclusion of all personnel working with the patient, helping agency in communities, in planning and decision-making, etc.
- Variety of persons involved and disciplines represented in most programs considerable effort may be made by staff in working towards mutually sharing relationships.

ORGANIZATION AND ADMINISTRATION OF PSYCHIATRIC UNIT IN A GENERAL HOSPITAL

There are some aspects of administration which influence implementation of concepts which are basic to occupational therapy. some examples here are which help to understand philosophy of administration of occupational therapy.

Occupational therapy administration tone is directly proportional to hospital culture tone which affects administration of these service to a great extent. Its success is on the framework of administrative procedures and organizational frame.

The attitudinal tone flares can be seen for patients, associates in department/hospital, oneself, one's professional competence.

Therapeutic milieu and mental health processes are not exclusive of departmental organization and function. Recognize basic human needs as vital to administration, hence value of administration is great.

CHAPTER 27

Utilization of Activities

Activities give opportunity to express—Attitudes, Feeling, Ideation, etc. at nonverbal level can be considerable value in psychotherapeutic process and to understand unconscious of the patient.

Utilization of activities is to attempt to translate some of the theoretic concepts of object relationship into more concrete practical application to integrate these concepts better.

Psychic-phenomenon is high degree of unpredictability and do not readily lend themselves to measurement. The difficulties of living cannot be isolated from one other, as there is no clear cut functional boundary separating. For example, patient's self-concept, his sensory perceptions and his narcissistic needs. Personality and pathology have many variable and complexities.

SELF-CONCEPT AND IDENTITY

The nature of one's self-concept and personality identity is determined by one's early interpersonal relationships with the significant adult. To the extent that such relationships have been unsatisfying, anxiety provoking, etc. ones self-concept and identity are distorted, confused, and/or inadequate.

SEXUAL IDENTIFICATION

Confusion about distortion of, or lack of sexual identification is of course part of the patient's difficulties in self- concepts and lack of ego maturation. Certain activities and objects in given culture and society have a masculine or feminine association.

INFANTILE ORAL AND ANAL NEED

For developing realistic self-concept and ego strength can occur only to the extent that one's primitive narcissistic needs are gratified. Occupational therapy offer opportunities to fulfill these needs through activities like sucking, drinking, eating, chewing and blowing and those that use excretory substitutes such as smearing or building with clay, paints or soil. Success will depend on exact required activity selection and patient becoming actively involved in such regressive behavior and therapist supports in regression as his needs show. Other activities less symbolic may change to preparation of food for self and others, caring and feeding animals or blowing musical instruments. Anal activities may be collecting and filing.

DEPENDENCY

Many patients infantilize the basic dependency need. This need is coupled with fear of such relationships and constant expectation of rejection and/or loss of the love object and the condition/state which is caused by such dichotomy.

HOSTILITY

Projected and introjected hostility are extremely frightening since such feelings are perceived as untimely destroying oneself or others (as in schizophrenics). Activities soft, nonresistive material, and nonprogressive performance, and above activities of oral and anal needs can be used. Nature of occupational therapy makes it possible to structure these situations as in hammering within a mould, batting a ball, sewing, or cutting to a line will help.

REALITY TESTING

Perceptiual vagueness makes it difficult to be sure of what is real and not real which manifests in self distortions and external world by confusion, impaired judgment, indecision and even disorganization. The need for shared reality is critical. Structural activities in occupational therapy provide reality testing since they offer sensory contact in a composition that is well defined.

Many activities provide opportunities for an agreement on the nature of reality because they have easily understood and accepted values and purposes.

COMMUNICATION

When verbal interaction and/or expression is difficult or impossible for the patient, need to give creative and structured activities in occupational therapy.

Creative arts uncover the unconscious and help patient to develop awareness to some of these problems.

CHAPTER 28

Epilepsy

Epilepsy is characterized by brief convulsive sizures and loss of consciousness. The epileptics whose fits are controlled by drugs or fits occur infrequently can live successful life outside hospital.

COMMUNITY PROBLEM

- Any job taken to come to no aim which is unaffected
- With whom he works, understands his mood and accepts his fit.

Inpatient department is necessary only when fits occur so frequently that are uncontrollable without heavy sedation or is associated with dementia or psychosis. Epileptics showing high degree of irritability, perversity (not doing what is told) and desire for attention. Desire may be fulfilled by meeting need and persistence shows obstacle for social adjustment.

Over excitement and stimulation produces a fit. Lessen drugs if waking hours are occupied gainfully in relaxing but absorbing activities. Change these activities as and when need arises.

AIMS OF OCCUPATIONAL THERAPY

Explore possibilities to settle patient outside hospital which depends on patient's response to treatment and social/environmental factors.

- When his fits are being controlled—Therapist should try to keep touch with patient without side life
- Maintain and improve his behavior standards
- Maintain good work habits
- Invalid attitude avoided in the patient
- Due to morbid scumming to fits—He may not be in a position to go back to his previous job therefore assess his abilities for other jobs for vocational training.

Possibility of job in other areas may be made known to patient only when therapist has assertained his absorption there for sure.

If hospitalized then full balanced life work, recreation and social interaction should be encouraged within institutional limits.

THERAPIST-PATIENT RELATIONSHIPS

- Therapist approaches to epileptic in firm and kind attitude
- Discourage showing favors
- Praise satisfactory work or behavior.

Attention desire may be fulfilled by giving charge/responsibility to him which is carried out with pride provided it is within patient's ability and commendation given for the same.

SOCIAL RELATIONSHIPS

- Place them in different groups so that temperamental difficulties of one do not affect the other
- Epileptics settle with less difficulty in mixed groups of long-stay cases
- Do not mix hysterics and epileptics together when placed with short stay (suffering from mind and body illness) psychotics or neurotics (suffering from nervous illness)
- As epileptics and hysterics both demand attention—Hysterics may simulate fits
- Neurotics accept epileptics by retaining their insight, sympathetically
- Therapist should not recognize antisocial behavior of these patients
- Explain to patient by taking him to side that he may mend his way to go back to group and mind business there
- Draw his (epileptics) attention to needs of other patients and cooperation gained to satisfy them.

EPILEPTIC FITS

Grand Mal

This type is more dramatic in appearance of fits and may not pass unnoticed in departmental activity.

Petit Mal

Observe more constantly as disturbance of consciousness is less dramatic and passes off unnoticed in general activity of the department.

See for clear, safe, nonedging area so that fall in a fit does not injure patient. Place cushion underhead in major fits and loosen any tight clothing. If there is warning sign before fit give gag (gauze) in the patients mouth—As folded hanky—Placed patients back teeth.

There is less injury in clonic phase, if limbs are supported properly. As clonus subsides, place patient's head to one side so saliva can drain and any obstruction in mouth can come out. Leave patient in comfortable position till recovers.

Guard patient from unguarded fires, dangerous machinery, boiling liquids. Make such precautions known to epileptics so that they can protect themselves from injury.

ACTIVITIES

- Wide range activities as intellect and aptitude vary like normal people
- Industrial work, ward work ward utility and departmental activities will be more or less like outside hospital activities so may be given
- Craft activities which are recreational in nature may be introduced
- Make radio, TV along with cultural activities available to them— Subject to their overstimulation
- Main good habits of good appearance and personality should be encouraged
- Women may do domestic activities which hold interest mostly
- Create atmosphere in a situation lest a fit should occur. Mental hospitals provide shelter to many cases but epileptic colonies give much greater freedom to them where they live with families.

CONTRAINDICATIONS

- Which involve constant noise, movements and flashing lights
- Which involve use of sharp tools or machinery with danger
- Activities which are dull, monotonous and require less concentration.

LIAISON

- Epileptics who can be employed, make a positive recommendation to employer for such case
- Occupational therapist contacts social worker and vocational counselor and employer for same
- Epileptics need permanent hospital care in some cases. So therapist must be kept informed of their progress in utility department of the hospital/sheltered workshop.

Hospitalization leading to fear and hopelessness

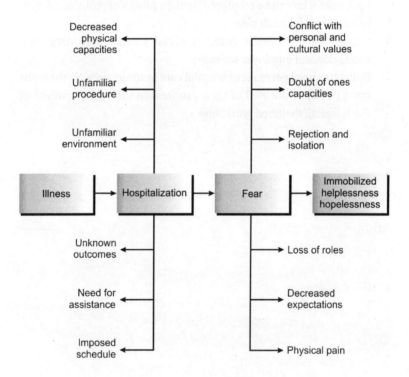

CHAPTER 30

Elements of
Occupational Therapy Process

INITIATION

- Referral and case finding
- Determination of services required
- Identification of strengths and deficits
- Goal setting.

METHODS AND PROCEDURES

Core Methods

- Therapist client relationship
- Selected activity to facilitate occupational performance
- Environmental manipulation and adaptation.

Additional Methods

- Psycho education
- Home programs
- Family instruction
- Specialized technologies.

OUTCOMES

- Development and restoration of occupations
- Improvement of maintenance of occupational function (rehabilitation)
- Improvement or maintenance of quality of life
- Stabilization and prevention.

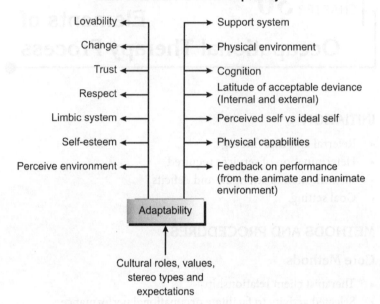

Elements that increase adaptibility

Lovability	Support system
Change	Physical environment
Trust	Cognition
Respect	Latitude of acceptable deviance (Internal and external)
Limbic system	Perceived self vs ideal self
Self-esteem	Physical capabilities
Perceive environment	Feedback on performance (from the animate and inanimate environment)

Adaptability

Cultural roles, values, stereo types and expectations

CHAPTER 31

Employment of the Disabled

Unemployment is common in disabled persons. It is partly due to ignorance of employers who employ disabled and disabled being work shirkers and due to employment allowances. It is very important role to get employed for life-time and helps in fulfilling the social role of the life-time. Work/employment provides economic security, intellectual or physical challenge and friendship helps to promote life satisfaction and helps in self-definition and estimating self-worth. Many view, work as an interruption in real life and others as a more meaning full life.

Work oriented disabled is always eager to participate in work intervention. Most disabled mourn their disabilities and thus like to work through process of determining abilities for work. They like to know where they should go for such services when they are ready. Though work has positive values yet many do not benefit due to disabilities.

Head injury disabled is severally affected with learning or appropriate social behavior problems. If unemployable due to any reasons he should be taught satisfying vocational persuits to enhance his quality of life.

The level of motivation is the greatest determining factor concerning return to work. Motivation is to a person's determination or persistence in persuing a goal. When no motivation exists or can be generated, the rehabilitation specialists must realize that work planning, evaluation and training will be unsuccessful. For those clients motivated by earning power and/or personal satisfaction, more opportunities than ever exist for employment. On going technological advances are providing significant employment opportunities for people with disabilities, including those individuals with severely limited physical abilities.

The job should fit a person's realistic self-image and values of work. Discussions during early phases of work rehabilitation, concerning work related issues, job versus career, pay versus personal satisfaction, office work versus physical work or small company or large—help the person not only to clarify his values but also to develop realistic attitudes and self perception.

The worker role interview—An instrument in its early phases of development, may be a useful tool in assisting occupational tharapists in identifying psychosocial and environmental variables associated with return to work.

Perhaps greater barrier to employment of people with disabilities is attitude. Sensitivity training is needed to assist co-workers and employers to overcome negative stereotypes of people with disabilities First we should understand who is disabled one who has a permanent or temporary physical or mental impairment that substantially limits one or more major life activities, e.g. walking, speaking, breathing, seeing, hearing, learning, caring for oneself or working. Substantially limits refers to the nature and severity of the disability, how long it will, or is expected to last, and its permanent or long term impact or has a record of such an impairment, e.g. a h/o cancer or heart disease even if cured, controlled or in remission or is regarded as having such an impairment, e.g. a person who is treated as if he or she had AIDS.

Determining essential functions of a job is a task that occupational therapist may perform. If this is the case, it is important to keep in mind that in identifying an essential function, therapist should focus on the purpose of the function and the result to be accomplished rather than the manner in which the function presently performed. For example, for a job requires a computer, the 'Essential Function' would be the ability to input, access and retrieve information from a computer not necessarily the ability to finger the keyboard or to see the monitor.

Reasonable accommodations include modifications in the work environment or in the way work is customarily performed that enable an individual with a disability to enjoy equal employment opportunities. For example, it means restructuring job, adjusting a work schedule to meet an individual's needs, adapting equipment or providing a reader or interpreter. Undue hardship is not granted to business.

Occupational therapist have a great role to play to improve hiring practices, the occupational therapist must structure employee job descriptions in terms of functional performance of specific tasks. occupational therapists offer services to people with disabilities who need to establish or reestablish salable skills and abilities and to the injured worker to restore function and to recover capacities needed to return to the job. Occupational therapists give service to normals also to prevent injuries or illness at work place and to help those clients who are displaced or retired early from work to reestablish their sense of productivity and worth.

To plan efficient return to work of a client, OT needs to be current on local, state and Government—level rules and regulations and the expectations of the workers compensation policies.

"Obtain a comprehensive history of the individual's occupational performance related to activities of daily living, work and play/leisure and identify the individuals work related behaviors, interest, abilities, needs and goals. Assess the sensory motor, cognitive, and psychological skills and deficits of the worker and potential worker while considering his or her future goals. Analyze resources, constraints, demands and expectations in the home, school, work site or community environment of the worker or potential worker to facilitate progress towards identified goals.

The ideal goal is injury or disability preventation. Most of the workers are at risk of back injury or cumulative trauma disorders of the hand and wrist. Musculoskeletal injuries are very common. Low back pain is the major cause of disability.

On site comprehensive work analysis is must.

ERGONOMIC WORK SITE ANALYSIS

This analysis is done to classify jobs according to the qualifications and physical demands that they require to determine whether or not an individual is capable of safely doing the job. It also helps to analyze whether disabled can go back to job or can apply for specific new job and to prevent work place injuries, such as biomechanical cumulative trauma disorders of employed workers. The term ergonomics or human factors refers to the characteristics of people that must be considered when arranging tools and equipment so that the job can be performed effectively and safely. The science and techniques of ergonomics are used to determine whether or not certain work activity causes an observed incidence of cumulative trauma disorders. Procedure has three facts:

1. A structured oral interview to identify the worker's perception of hazards and sources of physical discomfort
2. Screening for impairments and functional limitations—Including measures of sensation, strength and range of motion to obtain
3. A cleaner and clearer picture of nature and severity of health complaints.

There are many work site analysis forms drawn by various occupational therapists as per their experience and needs.

Ergonomic analysis are confined to three major areas: Work methods, work station design and worker posture, and handle and tool design. The work method analysis is concerned with determining what the worker must do to perform the task successfully, which requires direct observation or videotaping of the worker, counting the number of repetitive movements in a given work cycle and measuring or estimating the forces required by the job. The amount of time that the extremity is maintained in a certain stressful posture is important to note (that) because the stress on the structure accumulates. Also considered are the speed, intensity and pace at which the worker must perform repetitive movements to meet production standards.

EDUCATION AND TRAINING

Occupational therapists usually provide education and training program that are job specific rather than generalized principles.

Many educational and training programs provided by occupational therapists involve demonstrative and practice of biomechanically correct techniques that were first presented to the workers via lecture and discussion. Such programs may also include feedback to the workers at the work site and positive reinforcement regarding the use of body machincs and safe work postures. Coaching is typically on site with follow-up provided to managers and supervisors provided so that safe work habits are continually reinforced.

Work site health promotion should also be provided by occupational therapists wellness is perceived as a dynamic way of life in which good health habits are incorporated into one's lifestyle to improve both health and the quality of life.

Work assessments begin the rehabilitation process for injured on job workers which should develop to work hardening gradually.

FUNCTIONAL CAPACITY EVALUATION

It may include test of manual material capabilities, aerobic capacity, postures mobility tolerance, anthropometric measurements, ADL, energy conservation techniques and need for adaptive methods or technology.

PHYSICAL CAPACITY EVALUATION

It consists of assessment in isolation of parts of the body of functional units, e.g. lumbar region. In some return to work programs high instrumentation is used, e.g. cyber sagittal strength devise.

The smith physical revaluation is used by many occupational therapists in USA. It has 154 performance items and was found to be 86.5 percent accurate in predicting reemployment of workers with physical disabilities.

WORK CAPACITY EVALUATION

Residual physical disability requires the person to either change this type of employment or to resume previous employment using adapted tools or methods. In either case, the person's ability to work safely and efficiently must be determined. It is a comprehensive process that systematically uses work, real or simulated to assess and measure an individual's physical abilities to work. Practical, reality based assessment are used to evaluate work abilities related to specific job tasks.

Primary evaluation factors are those that comprise general "work ability", i.e. employment feasibility and work tolerance. Feasibility concerns with those basic factors that affect work acceptability to an employer in the labor market. Work productivity, safety and interpersonal behavior. It functions as gate keeper to triage clients into those who are able and unable to benefit from the vocational rehabilitation (Program) process and for others pre vocational services help to optimize their work potential. Certificates can be issued later.

On the job and work site evaluations are also important.

• Situational assessments also help
• Psychometric instruments are also used
• Interventions of OT/PT/Voc. Councillor/psychologists
• Work hardening is work oriented treatment and outcome is measured.

TYPES OF EMPLOYMENT

Supported employment: Offers paid work in integrated community with permanent follow along or supervision to citizens with severe disabilities. It is a job placement and training approach intended for persons who have been traditionally ineligible for otherwise vocational rehabilitation services because of their need for continuing support to maintain a job.

In 1980, some strides have been made towards supported employment and there is now an abundant effort in this direction.

Mentally retardeds with moderate, severe or profound range 1Q < 55 or have severe or multiple physical or sensory handicaps, autism, severe traumatic brain injury or history of (h/o) chronic mental illness are for such employment.

General supportive employment criteria is funds for such mentally retarders who traditionally not eligible for rehabilitation services and must have ongoing support for duration of employment.

Such persons should have individualized work supported rehabilitation plan reflecting ongoing support from other areas also.

Person must average 20 hrs/week over the course of his or her normal pay period.

Not more than 8 persons will be at a support employment work site.

No worker with handicapping conditions must be able to have regular contact with people who do not have disabilities, other than personnel providing support services while at the job site.

Competitive wage should be paid with proper labor standards.

A state rehabilitation agency can provide funding for supported employment for upto 18 months or as per government rules beginning at the time of placement.

Individual and except those with chronic mental illness, need as part of their ongoing services job skill training at least twice monthly.

Those with measured 1Q <40 and poor social skills fall in this category.

Barriers for finding employment related to job performance are:

- Behaviors exhibitory self-stimulation
- Self abuse
- Inappropriate verbalizations
- Lack of some daily living
- Personal care skills
- Independent eating and appropriate grooming skills
- Lack of functional language
- Reading skills and mathematical skills
- Cannot move about independently in the community without direct instruction
- Handicapping conditions as autism, deafness, blindness and cerebral palsy (CP).

CRITICAL EMPLOYMENT VARIABLES

- Meaning and value of work
- Supported employment regulations
- Staff members
- Transition and interagency coordination
- Integration
- Training in skills other than those specifically related to job performance
- Transportation

- Funding constraints and economic disincentives
- Applied behavior analysis
- Variety of work environment
- Job development and modification techniques
- Alternative job support strategies
- Appropriate schemesh for vocational training programs
- Family involvement
- Open employment/sheltered employment.

PREVOCATIONAL SKILLS

To develop prevocational skills, a detailed evaluation of the case is needed to identify and emphasize simple tasks, such as sorting and folding liner or clothing, task attendance and completion and clearing of the work area at the end of the anising a session. Specific skills that are useful in a vocational setting, the difficulty with such specificity of training lies in determining future placements of specific individuals.

CHAPTER 32

Psychiatric Occupational Therapy

Occupational therapy in a psychiatric hospital has certain general aims which relate broadly to every patient. These are:

1. Distraction from or acceptance of morbid Preoccupation. The patient cannot be distracted from his symptoms unless he is prepared at least to some degree, to cooperate. In order to gain his attention, the environment must attract him in some way. Activity in line with the patient's conscious interests and likely to use his intellectual capacity to the full, without (previous) overtaxing him or producing anxiety, may appeal. How this may be achieved is discussed. The approach may have to be less direct, more varied and with less expectations of the normal response than would be anticipated from a patient who is physically ill.

2. Deflection and/or diversion of drives: The use of energy creatively or its modification in such a way that the patient is enabled to live more normal life than he could if his impulse were allowed direct expression, is of vital importance. Drives may be expressed in aggressive, destructive or other psychopathological behavior. Energy which might otherwise be used destructively may be given socially acceptable expression in learning rags for stuffing toys made by other patients, by wedging clay to be used in modeling, tearing paper for paper mache. In each of these occupations the destructive activity proceeds a creative one even if the patient himself does not undertake the latter. Sharing in the work of another, he may however, begin to learn the rudiments of cooperation.

PREVENTION OF PROGRESSIVE

(a) Intellectual (b) Personality Impairment.

Intellectual

By providing activities which are within his intellect encourage a patient to use, his intellectual capacity, an attempt is made to prevent intellectual impairment. In melancholia, e.g. an attack is made on the symptoms of the patient, the occupational therapist attempts to interest and occupy him so that he attends fully his work or recreational and exercises his intelligence over it. By this means, he may be deflected from pre occupations and delusions. In such cases, the patients intellectual functioning can return to normal once he is symptom free.

The patient suffering from organic brain disease may be deteriorating initially. This process will be irreversible. The patient should be occupied to the highest intellectual level of which he is capable, remembering the deterioration does not take place in an unwavering decending curve but fluctuates. The main principles are to teach the patient, skills and techniques which become habitual through over learning, so that if the patient's condition worsens, he can continue working, although incapable of learning other process of similar difficulty. Normal personal and social habits should also be reinforced.

It is important to the occupational therapist to know the results of the intelligence tests of the patients, for once the intellectually impaired patients are symptom free, he may be able to return to his previous job unless it is contraindicated for some other reason. This is the case with most psychoneurotic patients.

The patients who is becoming progressively impaired or deteriorated, however will present a different picture, since the prognosis in his case will not be so good. A degree of normal living may be achieved, if habit training is started early, and if use is made of remaining abilities and of the fluctuations in the patients mental state. Nursing care may be minimized and the patient's interest in life prolonged by a well planned program of treatment.

Shapiro contends that psychomotor slowness underlies poor performance in cognitive task involving vocabulary problem solving and memory for new facts. When his slowness was kept constant there was no significant difference in ability shown by groups of psychoneurotic and psychotic patients whose illnesses were of long standing. This suggests that one of the most important aspect of treatment of the chronic psychotic should be to "speed him up". It is possible that craft work allows the patient to work too slowly for his own good and, as suggested elsewhere some psychotics may gain greater benefit from recreations or other occupations in which by nature of the activity itself, they are force into reacting more quickly than they would do in less demanding circumstances.

PERSONALITY IMPAIRMENT

Personality impairment may be characterized by disorganization of traits or by over. Organization, rigidity and failure to adapt to new circumstances. It cannot be considered apart from cognitive impairment and is intimately related to the whole treatment of the patient in the occupational therapy deptartment and elsewhere. The occupational therapist may find considerable difficulty in achieving report with patient whose personality is so disorganized that their communications are grossly distorted or incomprehensible or where the patient misconceives and distorts the situation to fit his delusional pattern, or where he suffers from aphasia. Although the illness from which the patient suffers must never be forgotten, it is neverthless a unique personality which suffers the illness. For this reason and for the reasons given above it is essential that the occupational therapy department should provide, not only a secure environment and one in which the patient feels accepted but one in which a number of varying personalities can find interest. These interests should not only appeal to present needs but also allow for cultural development.

MAINTENANCE OF THE NORMAL PERSONAL, SOCIAL AND WORK HABITS

The general health and normal function of the patient will not be restored unless personal, social and work habits are maintained. The patient's day must be so organized, therefore that these habits are exercised, where they do not do so voluntarily, patients must be persuaded to care for their appearance. Women may be encouraged to have their hair cut or restyled, to adopt or renew the use of make-up and to take an interest in their clothes.

This may be done through demonstrations and dressmaking classes in the department. For patients who are more deteriorated, the habit training program being carried out in the occupational therapy department should relate to and reinforce that being carried out on the wards.

Social habits may be maintained through the day-to-day interchange in the department, itself, through the sharing of tools, the sharing of the group project, the making and handing round of tea at break times, etc. Activities including dances, dramatic production and the running of the club for themselves with minimal supervision, help the pateints to re-learn, or experiment with, various forms of social behavior. All psychiatric illnesses involves a failure in social adaptations to varying degrees.

The psychiatric patients have often failed to find or maintain his social context and have become solitary for one reason or another. Thus activities are not always understood or approved by his social groups but he may not care that this is so. Nevertheless a setting must be provided in which he can readjust himself with minimum of the strain.

Many patients find difficulty in making an appropriate adjustment to the opposite sex. A less one-sided view of the opposite sex will be fostered if patients work and learn together instead of meeting solely under the more superficial and perhaps more "glamorized" conditions of the dances, games evenings and other social functions of the hospital or pateint's club.

Work habits should be reinforced as soon as the patient is well enough to attend the simplest task. In the last resort, however, it is the patient who determines whether or not he will occupy himself. For this reason, it is extremely important that he should find his work congenial. Harding suggests that fully satisfactory social context for their activities includes for most people, the opportunity of immediate contact with others whom they know and like, a recognized function in their group and a sense of having the sanction of companions for a wide range of their own individual values. Work habits cannot be cultivated in a vacuum. The patient must first know and like the therapist, there must be a gradual introduction to other people with whom he will feel at ease, and the work given must appear socially relevant to himself and his community. He must also feel that what he thinks and does in other respects is acceptable.

In doing an occupation its own sake the patient may come to value the companionship and sanction of others, or the permissive atmosphere and the greater tolerance of idiosyncrasy within the hospital may make him sufficiently secure to be willing to try to work again. Once he is willing to accept responsibility, his work may be increased gradually in length of time and in comlexity, but always in relation to his mental and physical state and to the other treatments which he is undergoing.

The occupational therapy department should provide means where by the patient begins to look towards a return to work. When he has recovered from the stage of acute illness, he should be observed for a period, and his work tolerance, abilities and interests estimated. If the patient no longer needs some form of specific Rx, work in one of the hospital utility department or industrial schemes may provide an environment more akin to his previous job than the OT Deptartment. Men who have worked on farms, in grocery, stores, as cobblers, gardeners, painters, etc. can renew these skills and train up to a full day work. They will then tend to leave the hospital secure in the knowledge that previous abilities are not lost and new techniques may have been learned. They will know before they start to seek employment that they are employable, will be less likely to spend the first week in their jobs apprehensive lest they should appear out of practice.

For women, work in laundry/kitchen, stores, sewing room, doing typing in the department or helping in the library, may give confidence in the ability to return to work. Some departments of mental hospitals are now equipped with kitchens, where patients may have demonstrations and lectures in cooking and house hold management. In many cases this may be extremely helpful, but it should be remembered their ability to run a home is not usually a primary cause of breakdown, but is more likely to be a symptom. Not all women therefore, will benefit from this instruction. Many are, in any case, over-conscientous as regards their housework and housekeeping and leave themseleves insufficient time or energy for other creative and recreational persuits.

In an age of small family units, in which, each home is largely independent of others some women may feel cut-off from outside society and interests. For this reason, it might be more therapeutic for some patients to lower the level of their domestic aspirations and raise that of their intellectual and imaginative ones, through activities or courses run in the hospital itself or introduced by outside specialists or correspondence courses.

ENCOURAGEMENT OF THOSE ASPECTS OF PERSONALITY WHICH MILITATE AGAINST FUTURE BREAKDOWN

This is an important function of OT, the patient is thereby helped to adjust to his illness or to tolerate or overcome residual disability. Apart from the main diagnosis, patients may suffer from particular inadequacies and personality defects which tend to make them unhappy and difficult in their relations with others or which antagonize other people. They may feel unable to accept any role in which they do not get most of the attention and may be resentful if they cannot have their own way. A male patient may be overbearing in his relations with women. A women may seek to escape responsibility by the exercise of charm. Other patients may be unwilling to accept any situation which involves a feeling of gratitude to others. Some (may) will irritate by being ingratiating, causing a withdrawal of those whom they are most anxious to please. Untreated, these personality dysfunctions militate against successful adaptation to life after discharge.

The value in many group projects lies in the fact that the patients can, in part, re-educate each other. Where the psychotherapist is attempting to help the patient to modify his attitudes, the patient himself may try out new roles and responses to others and to some extent the environment can be manipulated to serve these purposes. In the group the patient can assess himself in relation to others and through this may be helped towards an objective appraisal of his personality.

COMBATING THE PROBLEM OF LONG HOSPITALIZATION

In considering the chronic patients, the student frequently resorts to a steriotype of a demand patient. It must be stressed that not all patients dement and that many paranoid patients who have the interest, may be taught skills to a very high level of efficiency. Such patients have longer in which to perfect their skills than neurotic patient and for them care of the library, book-binding, weaving for hospital use or sale, may take the place of a formal occupation. In such cases constant changes in occupation may be a disadvantage. Too often, it is assumed that the chronic patient is only capable of appreciating simple forums of entertainment, and that almost all cultural and individual activities are beyond him. It is important that the chronic patient should feel of use and participation in hospital industries may help to give him his satisfaction quite apart from his other therapeutic and economic considerations. Nevertheless, chronic and acute patients have sometimes felt that they are source of cheap labor, or they may hold that if they are too ill to work outside the hospital, they are not well enough to do so within it.

Misunderstanding can be avoided if the placing of each patient is given really careful consideration by several members of the rehabilitation team and if, where possible, the scheme of community life in the hospital is explained to the patient. The occupational therapist should know for herself what skills are involved in laundry and kitchen work, in store keeping and gardening as practiced in the hospital in which she works.

She should know the heads of those departments, be aware of their difficulties and develop a relationship in which have advise on placing patients in, not only accepted but appreciated. It is important to realize that one can only behave rationally where there is an opportunity to do so, i.e. where there is an element of choice and where there are decisions to be made. Where all that if the patient is unreserved, acceptance of his environment there can be no very high standard of volitional behavior. The occupational therapist must, therefore, bear in mind the relative values of "habit training", "total push" or more permissive approach, in considering individual treatment. She must also know something of the effects of current psychological, physical, and surgical treatments and their significance in occupational therapist.

As a result, both of the mental health Act of 1959 and of the increased use of chemotherapy, there is a marked tendency for long life and chronic patients to have a number of short admissions instead of one long admission. This can affect the planning of the patient's occupation to a great extent as the stress is very much on a quick return to home and work. With mobilization and the maintenance of interest and skills replacing the need for long-term occupational planning.

CHAPTER 33

Community Care

INTRODUCTION—THE BURDEN OF MENTAL DISORDER

The term mental disorder covers a wide range of conditions which share in common an experience of psychological distress and social dysfunctioning, either by the affected person, or those around him, or both. On one end are syndromes, which are definitely due to neurochemical imbalances or structural changes in the nervous system. Schizophrenia, Bipolar mood disorders, Dementias and certain categories of mental retardation come under this category. There is sufficient evidence that at least 2 percent of the population, whether in the industrialized nations or in the developing countries, whether in urban or in rural conditions, suffer from the effect of these illnesses. While a number can be treated or managed with appropriate medication, at least one-third end up with chronic disability needing financial and social support for their existence.

At the other end are conditions, which reflect a breakdown of vulnerable persons in response to environmental stresses. Anxiety, depression, vague somatic symptoms are examples in this category. It is estimated that 8 to 10 percent of population suffers from these conditions. Poverty and hunger are perhaps the biggest stressors. So is being a woman, or a member of lower castes, in hierarchical societies like India. Increasing urbanization and dislocation, which are directly related to economic development programs in poor countries, are other social stressors. There are enough research studies linking these factors with mental ill health, well summarized by Patel (forthcoming). There is also evidence that suicide rates, which are arguably the clearest indicators of mental stress, are high in India and constantly rising (Shah 1996).

Closely related to these stress—Related psychological disorders are conditions like alcohol and substance abuse which are the resultants of a complex interaction between stress related demand, government promoted supply (in case of alcohol which brings excise revenue) and criminal promotion (for other drugs, which are banned). Here, psychopathology merges with sociopathology.

The rates of alcohol consumption and alcohol addition of course vary across the country and the rates of alcohol dependence vary from 1 to 15 percent (ICMR-CAR CMH 1990) to 15 to 20 percent (Bang and Bang 1990). According to one report, the rates of alcohol consumption are rising by 15 percent per annum.

According to a World Bank report, 8.1 of the DALYS—A DALY being the disability adjusted life years, which is a measure of burden produced by specific disease—are lost due to mental disorder. This burden seems to be equal to, if not more than, that produced by diseases like tuberculosis, cancer and heart disease. Another 34 percent of the DALYS are lost due to such physical diseases where behavior related factors play a part, e.g. heart disease, lung cancer and sexually transmitted diseases.

CARE OF THE MENTALLY ILL

There was no tradition of institutional treatment for mental disorder before allopathic medicine entered India with the Europeans. The first mention of a mental asylum is in the records of Bombay Presidency 1745 to 46 (Weiss 1983). The number of mental hospitals was nineteen at the time of Independence. It has currently risen to 45 with a bed occupancy of 21,147 (Central Bureau of Health Intelligence 1992). The condition in these hospitals is, on the average, very poor. Except for a few, which can be counted on the fingers of the hand, most institutions are poorly staffed, poorly resourced and poorly motivated. The food, clothing and living conditions are abysmal. As recently as 1999, a workshop was held in NIMHANS, in Bengaluru, to address the problems of these institutions and to issue some recommendations (NIMHANS report 2000).

Early in the 1960s and 70s it was beginning to be realized that long-term institutional care of all the needy mentally ill was neither possible nor desirable. The answer was deinstitutionalization and community care. The following paragraphs describe the story of how the experiments in community care of the mentally ill have proceeded, during with discussion of issues, which still need to be tackled.

Fifty years ago, if someone had talked of community based programs for mental health care, he would have been considered over ambitious. At that time, the best we could hope for was compassionate custodial care within the four walls of a mental asylum. These ill people were left there, often for life, by their relatives and community, who would then forget about them. It says a lot for the progress made over the years, even in our country, that we talk not only of treating mentally ill patients in their own surroundings, but also of involving the community in preventing as well as in promoting mental health.

Beginnings

It has become customary and quite rightly, to begin the story of community psychiatry in India with Dr Vidya Sagar (Kapur 1971) who in the late 1950s, started involving family members in the treatment of the mentally ill admitted to the Amritsar Mental Hospital. He did this for purely practical reasons, he had a 900 bedded hospital, which was extremely short staff. He put up army surplus tents within the precincts of the hospital, and the relatives who brought in new patients were requested to stay on to assist in providing nursing care.

Subsequently, when asked to analyze the impact of his innovation, Dr Vidya Sagar felt that the exercise achieved much more than he had initially hoped for. First, it reduced the hostility in the minds of the patients of having been abandoned in a strange place. Secondly, when the family started seeing the patients getting better, it helped to remove the age-old-myths about the incurability of mental illness. Finally, by taking group sessions, the relatives learnt the essential principles of mental health and were thus motivated towards improvement in their own ways of life. The involved were those who assisted Dr Vidya Sagar in this experiment. What they remembered most vividly was that many patients actually went back with their families and that the discharge statistics began to rise. All this happened before the era of major tranquillizers.

Tranquillizers

The entry of antipsychosomatic drugs in the late 1950s and early 1960s so dramatically controlled the agitation, aggression and withdrawal tendencies of the patients that it became possible to treat the mentally ill in general hospitals. Once again, those who were participant in the new revolution involved as was in setting up a general hospital psychiatric unit in a medical college hospital during the mid 1960s. What was most of the surprise of the other hospital patients that the mentally ill were in fact like other people and responded to medical treatment. Even more interesting were the new sense of confidence in psychiatrists and a visible rise of their status amongst their fellow professionals. More and more graduates started taking up psychiatry as a career. Currently, there are about 200 such units in the country (Murthy 1992).

Psychiatric Camps

The next logical step towards involvement of the community was the practice of holding psychiatric camps in remote villages (Kapur, et al, 1982). The reasons for holding such camps were the difficulty of taking patients to distant hospitals and the cost of travel. However, the main achievements of these camps were the involvement of community leaders and neighbors in the therapeutic process and reducing the stigma of mental illness. When one family was willing to have its sick member treated openly, it was easier for others to follow.

Further advances were the setting up, during the mid 1970s, of the National Institute of Mental Health and Neurological Sciences (NIMHANS) in Bengaluru and the Post Graduate Institute of Medical Education and Research (PGIMER) in Chandigarh, where there were programs to teach doctors and health workers in the primary health centers, the skills for early recognition and management of mental illness (Kapur 1979, WIG et al. 1981). The reasons for starting such programs were practical, the country just did not have, nor was likely to have for decades, the necessary specialist staff to deal with all its severely ill psychiatric patients. What these programs achieved, more than anything else, was the demystification of the phenomenon of mental illness. It was made obvious that a non-specialist doctor or a village health worker could do, after a short period of training, what previously only a highly trained specialist was expected to accomplish.

The success of these programs was internationally recognized and they were emulated elsewhere both within and outside the country. The demystification process was carried forward at NIMHANS where the community members have been trained to recognize and follow-up mentally ill patients (Ra et al. 1990). NIMHANS also adopted a district in Karnataka to further develop this program (NIMHANS Bulletin 1988). Parallel with the rural progress have been the developments in urban settings where general practitioners, school teachers and lay volunteers are being trained to recognize and manage mental illness (Sham Sunder et al. 1978, Kapur M, 1988). There is still the problem of numbers. With 2 percent of the population suffering from severe mental disorders a great amount of time, effort and money is needed to spread these programs across the country. However, this change which has taken just 40 years, has produced an upbeat feeling in the minds of mental health professionals. But the picture is not rosy.

Firstly, it has been discovered that while these training programs run well in research situations, when tested in unsupervised situation they do not do so well. One study (ICMR 1987) which aimed at testing the impact of training the PHCs then leaving them to detect and treat the patients, showed that in fact the results were poor, both with respect to recognition and management of the patients. The main cause of poor response was poor morale of PHC staff and their preoccupation with other vertical programs, like family planning.

Secondly, the success of such programs, in best of conditions, also depends on the support and care which the family can provide. One is not sure whether the families in a situation of fast social change can be depended upon to provide such support.

FAMILY AND THE CARE OF THE CHRONICALLY ILL

In the 1960s program was started in the USA and subsequently in other western countries to treat mentally ill patients outside mental hospitals. This program was started, not because there was a shortage of mental hospitals but because of the new knowledge, which showed that long-term hospital stays could lead to chronicity. The program involved the setting up of half-way homes, hostels and most importantly, the treatment of patients in their own family settings through follow-up visits by nurses and social workers. It was soon discovered that even rich western nations did not have sufficient funds to run the half-way homes and the domiciliary services. Above all, the family was just not willing to keep the patient. The result was that the patients were coming back to the hospitals through a kind of revolving door situation and if the readmission policy was strict, they became homeless and roamed the streets. As recently as 1985 a disturbed psychiatric patient was seen walking about parks around Harvard University and also read reports of patients who were violent on the streets and some who died of exposure. The first reaction was self-congratulatory. "Are we not so much better off in India where the family is willing to look after its own? This reaction was short lived because it was soon discovered that a western family was not so much unwilling, and unable to do the caring. With the nuclear family being the norm, all able bodied people going to work and children going to school, who would look after the patients during the day or even at night, following a hard day.

FAMILY CARE IN INDIA

The tide is turning in India as well. There is an increasing migration to the cities, a gradual diminution of family size and fewer people available to stay at home to look after patients. Quite likely, even in India, that people will continue to look after the mentally sick when other pressures increase? The process of social change is going to become faster with the new economic philosophy. I am afraid that family support is not going to be easily available in the future and if, the community is interested in the welfare of the mentally ill, it will have to think of other means.

The writing is already on the wall. Wherever half-way homes for the chronic mental patient are available, they are running full and have long waiting lists. This, in spite of the fact the most places charge amounts which are more than the annual incomes of average India families. As I worry about this, I am appalled that almost all the mental hospitals of the country are vying with each other to give up their asylum function the shorter the stay of the patient in the hospital, the more modern and scientific they are supposed to be. The space and services, which were reserved for chronic patients in the old fashioned hospitals, are dwindling away rapidly.

Just as 20 years ago, when we started innovative programs for the treatment of the mentally ill, we must now start developing innovative programs for the care of the chronically mentally ill patients. Before accelerating social change forces the family to deposit its chronic patient on the road, we must start planning for a roof over his or her head and arrange food, clothing and some recreation, to put some meaning into his life. This is too big a task to be left to the private sector. In spite of all the effort in the last 10 years, there are only about 250 places for chronic mental patients in private establishments. The funds required for even for the minimal care of non-productive chronic mental patients are massive. The government will have to shoulder the responsibility and the planning process should start immediately. It is in this context that the giving up of the asylum function by the mental hospitals, which possess lot of space as well as a fair number of nursing aides, seems so irresponsible.

COMMON MENTAL DISORDERS

Epidemiologists will claim that while the prevalence rate of psychoses is 1 percent that of neuroses 8 to 10 percent. This is perhaps true but if we include conditions such as substance abuse and personality disorders of various kinds in this category, the percentage will be even higher. It is also true that at least one-third of the patients who go to nonpsychiatrists, suffer from psychological rather than physical illness. However, these conditions are not diseases in the usual sense of the term but an expression of their inability to cope with the difficulties of life. Most of these patients require psychotherapy and social intervention rather than medicines or surgery. Unfortunately, there has been an increasing medicalization of distress. The average doctor has neither the time nor the basic skills to deal with the stress, which has made the patient seek his help and finds it convenient to prescribe tranquillizers. These, of course, work only temporarily and if used for a long-time lead to dependence and abuse. What the patient needs is help in developing sensible coping strategies.

There was a time when society offered different kinds of support measures to the stressed, in the form of family elders, village mantarwadis (sorcerers) and temples. Stories from folklore and mythology were used to rouse a person to a meaningful existence in the face of life's trials. There were clear cut values to live by. Social change has diluted these values and the stories which were effective before, now appear to be naive and irrelevant. The situation is much worse in urban slums where the sense of alienation is even greater and social support less. What kind of community effort is needed to devise new social values and supportive links? Tranquillizers are not the answer and what we need urgently is an effective community education program to fight the excessive use of these drugs. We must also focus on the drug company general practitioner axis and counter the pressure that the companies exert to prescribe their medicines, a pressure which is in the form of subtle and not so subtle inducements.

ROLE OF THE MASS MEDIA

The media can obviously play a big role in the management of mental illness, but unfortunately what one often sees behind an exercise is an attempt to titillate and shock at the cost of someone else's emotional pain. Education about mental health is a task of great responsibility and before anything else, media persons who undertake this should themselves learn about the complexity of the human mind and the multifactorial nature of emotional disorders. What is required is a sacred partnership between professions and media persons, each giving and receiving an accurate feedback on this sensitive issue.

The promotion of mental health is too important a matter to be left to mental health professionals alone. There is a lot in our spiritual heritage as well as in textbooks of psychology which shows that faith and a life style compassionate to others can increase out stress tolerance. There is also evidence that consistent parenting and a schooling which provides meaningful challenges, without oppressing the child, can prevent the occurrence of mental disorders in later years (Kellam 1994). These principles strike at the very root of the civilization, which we see today—A civilization, which is built on the edifice of greed and competition of power. Will this civilization destroy itself? We can see the difficulties involved when plans to cut down the depiction of sex and violence on the cinema and television screens meet with resistance, even when there is fairly conclusive evidence that symbolic violence of this kind promotes real life violence (Newson 1994). Good wishes and education programs are not enough; we need firm political action.

CHAPTER 34 Occupational Therapy in Mental Subnormality

DEFINITION

What is MR? The Random House Dictionary of English Language refers it as to the term "Mental Deficiency" which it defines as lack of some mental power or powers associated with normal intellectual development resulting in an inability of the individual to function fully or adequately in everyday life.

It does not differ much from American definition of American Association on Mental Deficiency (AAMD). MR refers to significantly subaverage general intellectual functioning existing cocurrently with deficits in adaptive behavior and manifested during the developmental period.

Its apparent frank definitions that the MR do not demonstrate only one area of difficulty but do, indeed, manifest an interaction of multiple factors including, sociocultural, psychological and physical influences.

HISTORY OF MENTAL RETARDATION (HISTORICAL PERSPECTIVE)

The historical review provides an understanding of the specialty area of MR as well as the motivating forces of those currently involved with planning and demanding accountability.

PERCEPTUAL DEVELOPMENT

When sensation is registered in the brain, the child, must derive meaning from it. This is accomplished by relating the current experience to learning that has already occurred. Thus, the child can perceive the ball as part of a game because he or she has already had experience with round objects that are thrown. Over the time, child builds up (reparative) of knowledge about the world that is based on visual, auditory, motor and cognitive perceptions. The child explores new things, reaches them on basis of earlier experience and modifies his or her existing concepts while integrating the new experience into an old scheme.

HISTORY OF OT IN MENTAL SUBNORMALITY

The historical studies provide an understanding of the speciality area of mental retardation as well as the motivating forces of those currently involved with planning and demanding accountability.

History tells us that earlier mentally subnormals were ignored or received little or no attention and care. They were placed in woods to (act to avoid) fend themselves or die. Life for average person was ardous so for who needed extra care it was not possible. The other reason for desertion was that they were possessed by the Demons.

During middle ages, the role of the court jester was usually filled by retarded person. The observations now show these were Down's Syndrome cases. When these lived with parents and families, filled the role of "Village Idiot."

Those who fill role today, they run errands, carry messages for small tip for self-satisfaction and worth to gain social acceptance.

Various religious orders became so distressed with lack of physical care, the redi.cule, and abuse given the retarded that sheltered communities were built. With these kindly isolation sense of hopelessness grew. The good care and shelter was not sufficient for little mental stimulation, this resulted in regression and deterioration.

In 1800s, Jean Itard, a physician working with deaf got involved in a 12-year-old boy whom he caught in the forests of Aveyron, France, a diagnosed case of Mentally subnormal by Pinel who was an associate of Itard. Understanding that intellectual performance and potential could be affected by environmental stimulation and opportunity, Itard started working with sensory motor techniques to achieve the goals.

Initially, he started working with Victor through the sense of hearing. After occluding visual stimuli, Victor fired with auditory stimuli and required an affected response. Nest discrimination in noises he proceeded in verbal clues. The blindfold was removed quickly to request to rule out extraneous visual distractions. Itard then concluded that Victor was lowering the importance of visual stimuli—Most frequently used and highly sophisticated sense.

When Victor responded to sense of anger, sadness and happiness in vocalizations, Itard proceeded to the sense of touch and under similar proceeding to sense of smell and taste. This was a promising sequence of training. This was discarded for sometime but was resumed in 1900s. Though MRs could not be fitted into the society but were a great help to evolve an effective attitudinal change regarding the mentally retarded.

Seguin, a student of Itard, modified on Itard's work and developed what he called the "Physiological Method" of training. After coming to USA, he opened residential fascilities for MRs and his involvement led to American Association of Mental Deficiency (AAMD).

Like other specialty areas, the unqualified persons promised cures which they could not effect as mental retardation is incurable which caused reversal of feelings in the minds of people about their (MRs) potential of work in mentally retarded negating work of Itard and Sequin resulting into hopelessness.

This futility attitude continued with the development of larger residential facilities in isolated areas. Society was getting convinced that facilities for mentally retarded are being created.

By the end of World War II, emphasis shifted and came to include programing by the National Association of Retarded Citizens (NARC), an organization by the parents of mentally retarded persons and interested lay persons.

It was for the first time that the professionals were accountable for both resultant behavioral changes and utilization of funds.

Due to lengthy litigation between the commonwealth of Pennysylvania and parents regarding educational facilities available, a Right to Education concent Agreement was implemented in 1973. This guarantees educational facilities to mentally retarded and physically handicapped children to an age of 21 years. This was a major accomplishment of parents of mentally retarded. Other states studied the agreement for implementation.

The public law 94 to 142 the education for all handicapped children Act came into being in 1975 after Federal Government passed it. The major effect of this act on occupational therapy is that all special education programs will have occupational therapy/psychotherapy available either on staff or as an consultant by Sept, 77.

A positive change was seen now in all training centers. Funds were not able to effect change. Society treated mentally retarded as isolated/institutionalized cases for custodial care.

Professionals had not assumed responsibility for preparation to work with mentally retarded pressures, NARC forced accountability on professionals in care of mentally retarded.

The training is now being imparted to have open, zealous, conscious people willing to work for welfare of mentally retarded from training schools, centers, institutions.

OCCUPATIONAL THERAPY IN MENTAL RETARDATION

General objectives of OT in mental retardation are:
  i.   It should be long term OT Planning.
  ii. Treatment program and consideration of problems should be separate for each patient.
  iii. Greater part of the treatment of these children in respect of psychological needs and practical necessities should be carried out in large groups.
  iv. Avoid too much attention to avoid dependence.
  v.   Too much individual attention should be avoided to obtain desired results.
  vi. Encourage individual treatment initially but should be withdrawn gradually as the patient becomes absorbed into groups where he develops latent qualities of initiative or of leadership.
  vii. Make efforts to provide good environment and experiences as varied as possible to make atmosphere conducive to mental stimulation.

The specific treatment objectives may vary according to the extent of mental retardation.

SEVERELY MENTALLY SUBNORMAL

For the purpose of clarification this group has been divided into two subgroups.

1. Treatment for very severely subnormals aims at covering those who usually have IQ below 30 but includes those with slightly higher level as well.
2. Treatment for severely subnormal relates to those in the range of IQ between 30 and 50.

Very Severely Subnormals

1. Totally unemployable.
2. Entirely dependent on nursing care.
3. Apparently grossly physically abnormal or almost normal.
4. Have stunted growth.
5. Frequently assume huddled and crouching postures.
6. Apparently oblivious of their surroundings.
7. They wander, run about aimlessly or injure persistently.
8. Non-existent speech.
9. Word or phrase repeated like parrot again and again.
10. May show response to well known stimulus like sweet or dinner.
11. Do not attempt on construction of sentence.
12. Comprehensive of speech limited but not as verbal expression, tone of voice may convey more.
13. They are noisy, screaming grunting and croaking relating to various expressions.
14. They may be excited, destructive, spiteful and others may be duly passive.

Occupational Therapy Treatment

Treatment of such cases is a challenge to Occupational Therapist.

Aims in Training are:

a. Prevent deterioration.
b. Check habits harmful to themselves or others.
c. Assist in habit training routine.
d. Encourage purposeful activities.

e. Lessen dependence on others.
f. Direct activities on constructive channels.

To achieve above aims it is necessary to:

a. Gain their confidence and attract attention: Those who are too anxious show childishly and others unresponsive to any personal contract or variation to environment.
   - Use music with strong beat to attract their attention which will be exhibited by rocking movement which is encouraged to clapping or stamping.
b. Obtain interest and stimulate coordinated movements: Have variation in depth, rhythm and tempo of music. Musical games to develop competitive spirit. This is achieved after weeks/months and then develop to simple movements and exercises. Continue use of music to develop rhythmical and purposeful movements.
c. Develop and encourage purposeful movements: After obtaining large movements with gross muscle action—Slowly progress to small and finer movements through musical rhythm.

   The percussion band encourages useful stimulus to develop eye-hand coordination with organized group activities.

   More purposeful movements may be obtained by threading of cotton reels or beads and use of educational toys.
d. Useful Activities: Introduce employment of simple nature such as sand papering of wooden articles, threading off cuts of leather for window cleaners, tearing paper for paper mache.
e. Constructive activities: Simple craft activities which may be tried to inculcate good habits of work. May work in team with similar kind of work. Teach everyday skills some like lacing and tying shoe laces, manipulation of hooks and eyes. Apparatus used should be in same angle as an actual to be used.

   Each phase may take weeks or months but still the progress/results may not be visible.

OT program is governed by:

a. Adhere to routine of habit training and occupation.
b. Daily physical activities.
c. Carefully graduated occupations.
d. Persistent individual and group teaching.

Severely Subnormals

- Appearance small in stature
- Poor development with shambling gait
- Usually dress themselves.

OT Aims are

- Stimulate purposeful and coordinated movement
- Increase ability to concentrate
- Assess potential employment ability
- Teach some useful employment technique if possible
- Provide opportunity for social development.

Long-term planning and routine is important for this group of patients to establish good work habits. Plan systemic time table right from the outset. Break activity to simplest level so that concentration available is directed to a movement or sequence of movements within their capacity.

- Verbal instructions are of no use as speech is imperfectly understood
- Demonstrations are useful way to teach them which may be followed by patients own efforts as well
- Evoke tactile sense which is dull hence requires training to help guide limbs in the required movements
- Repetition helps to evoke such movements volitionally
- Present same set of materials in same circumstances to teach them through demonstrations with same key teaching words
- Slight change in sitting place may disproportionately disturb time
- This may be used by the therapist in overcoming temperamental disturbances
- Muscular coordination shall be helped by all kinds of simple physical activities
- Music may help in getting rhythmical and coordinated movements
- The games of competitive nature may help encourage individual effort
- If patient is allowed to sit without any activity it may affect finger movements to a great deal with manipulative power to nil
- Encourage constructive work as early as possible.

Introduce simple craft activity with following objects in view

a. To continue to improve concentration.
b. To increase manual dexterity.
c. To encourage methodical work habits.
d. To develop/instill feeling of confidence and joy of achievement inherent in the completion of a piece of creative work.
e. To help in the assessment of future employment potentialities.
   Next stage of treatment may be:
f. Training for specific employment within the hospital.
g. Training for processes of industrial type.
h. Further varied employment within the occupational therapy department for patients who may have good ability, but whose temperaments, preclude their employment in utility department.
i. A program of intensive training. In self-help and employment activities for patients who may return home, or be admitted to a local authority hostel.

MENTALLY SUBNORMAL

This group has IQ 50 or over. Physically may differ a little at all from normal. The immaturity may manifest from their dress and may be flamboyant in character with adornment at special occasions but uncared for and untidy in ordinary course of events. Many must have attended some schools or institutions where they must have picked up reading, writing, and making simple calculations. Speech may be defective to improper articulation. Difficulty in expressing ideas due to poor vocabulary although they can converse on the matter within their experience and comprehension of language also within same limits.

Intelligence in general may not be good but cannot make best use of it due to:

• Temperamental instability
• Social inadequacy
• Psychopathy.

OT Aims in such cases are

• Return to normal life of those who are capable of becoming self-supporting

- Return to their homes those who may be taught to adapt to family life, and perhaps make some contribution towards supporting themselves
- Help such patients as will always be needed/supportive care of the hospital or hostel environment to:
  - Become useful members of the hospital or hostel community
  - Take part in some kind of sheltered workshop scheme
  - Achieving proficiency in craft or other techniques with the object of upgrading to above statements.

GENERAL TREATMENT

Training to specific ends must rest on:

i. Security
ii. Self-confidence
iii. Good work habits.

Security: Instability in itself shows desire of security and stable existence which can be provided in OT by firm discipline and a quiet ordered atmosphere. Integrate in homogenous group to promote feeling of security and a desire for acceptance which aids socialization. Possess respect for staff who direct their activities with control and confidence. They loose confidence in staff who are argumentative with them.

The planned and ordered routine with quiet atmosphere and group relationship is probably the most important foundation of their training.

Self-confidence: Due to excessive overconfidence they ensure to meet life with equal terms and confidence—hence are withdrawn. Encourage personal appearance to develop self-confidence production of any work in OT creates a feeling of achievement and appreciation by others.

Good work habits: Future success in employment may depend on habits with points of

a. Concentration—Dependent on interest.
b. Perseverance—Dependent on incentive of a satisfactory goal.
c. Consistency—For good standard of work.

Encourage them to be critical of their own work which should be taught to strive for improvement. Criticize so that further effort is not discouraged.

SPECIFIC TRAINING

This can be planned on each case's
a. Ability
b. Intelligence
c. Initiative
d. Temperament
e. Home circumstances.

The planning can be in three stages

1. *The initial stage:* OT plays chief role at this stage and this should be a period of observation and assessment. Get to know the individual patients and forecast his abilities and social capabilities. Use any activities within department resources. They should cater for work, social and recreational needs.

2. *The intermediate stage:* Consider OT here as supportive and recreational stability at this stage which allows work in less sheltered conditions. Patients should work part time in institution, etc. Cookery and dress making classes for girls and woodwork and general utility classes for boys. Give education where academic abilities are present. Educational programs on TV may prove useful if any.

3. *The final stage:* At this stage OT takes educational and social form. This should provide normal way of living. Encourage employment on daily wages basis wherever possible.

From educational aspect, he should be prepared from day-to-day problems on entirely practical manner. Most patients are capable of the standards which are acceptable to employers outside.

For females special household training is necessary. They should be taught to plan their own meals with some regards for a balanced diet with limited budget—Allow them to make purchases from local shop, cook and prepare meals. Teach correct storing methods. Teach cleaning, use of modern labor saving equipments, etc.

PERSONAL APPEARANCE AND PERSONAL CLOTHES

Tips on washing and mending clothes will be useful. Teach hair styling, make-ups and grooming skills in general. Practice on public transport for traveling if need be. Use of public call infuses confidence in them. Instructions on seeking job and training. Arrange talks on above as much as possible.

The social activities can go to the extent of organizing functions themselves than to go to see a movie or dancing. Community life diminishes originality and initiative. Encourage, reading, gardening, hobbies, etc. Formation of social club which would help on various aspects of behvior.

So largely OT in mental retardation depends solely on teaching skills and personal drive of therapist. We may say that conscientious and energetic teaching, +ve enthusiasm, thoughtful choice of activity, can produce results in rehabilitation of these patients which are satisfying and surprising too.

Appendices

APPENDIX 1: PUBLIC PARTICIPATION AND INVOLVEMENT FOR ROAD SAFETY

Road safety is a habit. It is a culture which forms an integral part to be road worthy drivers along with vehicles. Taking care of oneself, thus for others is a curteous give and take amongst the road users. Road safety cannot be promoted with the man education approaches. We need to have mass education drills for the public in which later's involvement will be there. Some such measures and methods are listed below:

- Strict enforcement of traffic laws
- Group education sessions
- Creation of voluntary participation
- Footpath puppet shows
- One-to-one teaching of road safety rules
- Adaptation of a locality by volunteers to promote road safety.

Strict Enforcement of Traffic Laws

It must be done to ensure accident free roads as far as possible. High fines are very good deterrents to defaulters. These things educate the defaulters for future on laters' own cost. I will strongly advocate it in present times of financial crisis in the country. It should be observed strictly irrespective of any status of the defaulters.

The various fine ranges could be fixed which upon nature of the fault committed, defaulters are penalized. Under this defaulter will educate others also indirectly while narrating a date with traffic Police Officer after committing a fault.

Group Education Sessions

These can be arranged by the department with the help of local voluntary agencies working in the zone.

Say for example, an organization 'A' is selected where Traffic Police representative visits the place. Fixes up time and date with the head of the organization to show and teach various films/regulations of the department staff to the group employees of the agency. This agency may be asked in turn to educate another agency in the close collaboration of Road Safety Cell of Delhi Traffic Police.

Creation of Voluntary Participation

Here I would like to cite my own example.

It was about 10 years back that I got impressed of functioning of one DCP (Traffic) whom I did not know personally at all and also did not meet ever. Through the articles in newspapers, magazine, TV, radio-talks of that officer, I was impressed so much that I got motivated to associate myself a volunteer with this force.

I feel that even all others in chain after that officer had been the motivating force behind my continuing to be the voluntary force with the department till today. Here, one thing which comes to surface is that the doers also sometimes leave impact on the minds of the public men. Even one is motivated—the objective is achieved.

Footpath Puppet Shows

We know that theater has been an established media to convey message in its proper sense and spirit. The same could be exploited by Road Safety Cell of Delhi Traffic Police. This media has an advantage to attract people of any age. If in schools, the children become beneficiaries group, if in lunch time at a point where generally the people collect, sit, smoke, play cards and discuss politics, those will be the ripe points to stage such puppet shows. The people from Dance and Drama School, New Delhi could be associated with the staff of the department while formulation of scripts for such shows. Same way, the school children may be involved to act as puppets and convey various Rules/Regulations of Road Safety.

This is suggested because, It; has been seen in the past that when beneficiaries do not come forward we go to them to their door step. This is my message as a technologist.

One-to-One Teaching

This can be done in schools and colleges where preliminary education on Road Safety has been carried out The department can approach— the Secretary, Department of Education, Delhi Administration, to include Road Safety Education Program in socially useful productive (SUPW) in each school. This will mean that one school child will educate another child near his school or home on road safety rules. This will not only use child's time usefully and gainfully but also master the rules for oneself too. If It could be possible, that will go a long way to promote willing road safety learning amongst children.

Adoption of a Locality

The trained personnels in road safety could be asked to adopt a village/ locality near their residence—because going to far off places might cause inconvenience and lessen the spirit of social voluntary work.

With locally organized resources, the education and training in road safety could be promoted by Road Safety Cell of Delhi Traffic Police with the assistance of volunteers available with the department. Even volunteers from locality could be trained first as trainers who later impart training in road safety to fellow beings.

Apart from above, in other countries studies have shown that most injured in road accidents can be licensed as safe, competent drivers. Now even, lack of the essential medical input in commercial driving schools has kept many from succeeding.

While vehicles are purchased, the vehicle selling agencies must see for a driving license of the person concerned before other sale formalities are completed. As safety is drivers' concern first, he must be thoroughly trained before he is on the road with vehicle to avoid a killer on road side.

Most of the training of the public men should be carried out on the road so as to appreciate learned skills in driving:

There has to be a predriving evaluation of the driver's skills in the form of:

- Physical skills
- Perception
- Cognition
- Vision
- Language skills
- Need for adaptive driving equipment and vehicle modification.

This is essential for road safety requirements and road discipline. These should be fundamental prerequisite for any good driver to be. When driver equips him or herself, it is also a willing participation in upgradation of the driving skills. It has been said that about:

- 20 to 30 hours traning is needed for spinal cord injury
- 10 hours traning is needed for lower extremity amputations
- 10 hours traning is needed for CVAs
- 15 to 20 hours traning is needed for traumatic head injuries
- 20 hours traning is needed for congenital defects.

While concluding it can be summarized that participation and involvement of public is a "MUST" activity which must be undertaken by the department at all times to come in the future.

APPENDIX 2: DOCUMENTATION IN OCCUPATIONAL AND PHYSIOTHERAPY

Introduction

Document is an extremely effective tool for advocacy. It is often key to success when dealing with difficult situation. It calls for accountability and also allows for kudos when things go right.

It is your job to utilize tools that will enable you take carefully prepared documentation. You have written to the case presentation and read it aloud. This document be included as part of your parent input into the written records. Your document is written input which should hold equal weight with other information presented and considered at case conference/meeting/seminar/workshop or with other professionals of the case in respect of any patient.

It is being stressed for many years in health system, that proper documentation is very much needed by professionals of OT/PT giving a legal status to the patient care under their supervision. The same is stressed in consumer protection act (CPA) also.

Document what you and patient says, because it keeps the record clear without any misunderstanding. Verbal case handling must be documented after writing it in patient's case file with signatures and date.

Importance

1. Backbone of records in health care system.
2. Maintain records of patient if incorrect then it is malpractice, negligence.
3. Legal security if properly maintained.
4. Effective tool to preserve records.
5. Key to success for difficult situations.
6. Makes individual accountable.
7. Merit to keep proper records.
8. Input to account work and effort.
9. Credited towards excellent record keeping if meticulously done.
10. Maintain case clarity on treatment.

11. Maintain white actions.
12. Dated writing helps in legal cases.
13. Record of treatments/test/advised by treating therapist.
14. Properly documented records of patients settle legal cases fast.
15. Well documented records establish therapists credibility.
16. Proof of patient care.
17. Major treatment records.
18. Helps to record aspects of patient life.

History and Charting

The medically accepted guidelines are:
- Be factual, consistent and accurate
- Be written as soon as possible after an event has occurred, providing current information on the care and condition of the patient/client
- Not include abbreviations, jargon, meaningless phrases, irrelevant speculation and offensive, subjective statements
- Be accurately dated, timed and signed
- Be readable on photocopies (i.e. black ink)
- Be written, wherever possible, with the involvement of the patient/client
- Be written in terms that the patient/client can understand
- Be consecutive
- Identify problems that have arisen and action taken to rectify them.

Definitions

Documents are formatted information that can be accessed and used by a person. They have a beginning and an end and may be represented through alpha-numeric text, vector data, a digital map, spreadsheets and databases, moving images, or audio data. Regardless of format, documents serve the purpose of conveying information.

Records are documents that have been set aside as evidence and protected from alteration or change. The critical factor is how "set aside" is defined. In paper, "being set aside" means placing a document into a filing system from which it can be retrieved. With digital technologies, the same result is achieved by transferring an electronic document from an operational environment into a record keeping system.

Elements of a Record

Content is the information in a record, the idea or concept, the facts about an event, a person, an organization or other similar act that are recorded to document the transaction itself.

Structure refers to the physical and logical attributes of records. Physical attributes of a record include such things as the size and style of type, line spacing, page margins and agency logo. Logical attributes consist of the logical arrangement the record. For example, the structure of a memorandum would include a header (the name of the sender, the date, the subject of the memo and the recipient of the memo), a body (the actual content in one or more paragraphs) and the authentication (signature).

Context explains the "why" of the record. A single record derives its trustworthiness and usefulness from its association with other records that collectively tell the story of an event or activity.

Documentation in OT/PT

Definition

A written/printed paper furnishing information or evidence or a legal/official paper furnishing details of records.

Reasons

1. For administrative advice.
2. To maintain evidence.
3. To keep record.
4. To follow-up cases.
5. To conduct research.
6. To support legally.
7. To guide course of action.

8. To maintain authentic record.
9. To write progress notes.
10. To pursue case in future.

Purpose of Documentation

Cleave defined Record as a written statement to preserve memory and to present accurate evidence of acts and events.

Report is defined as written summary of facts or occurrence to communicate the information. As "progress report" and "discharge summary".

Documentation should be clear, easier, accurate, objective and complete.

OT/PT are responsible for keeping accurate records and writing appropriate records to document the treatment program and patients progress.

OT/PT have reduced documenting. OTs/PTs are required to improve writing skills that reflect objectivity, clinical accuracy, conciseness, completeness and a system of record keeping that is efficient.

Documentation is very very important part of OT/PT services and;

   i. Provides administrative control.
   ii. Complies with law and aids in litigation.
   iii. Provides, clear, objective data about the patient on which future treatment can be based.
   iv. Communicating progress to the physician or other health care professionals concerned.
   v. Provides justification for the records of the treatment.
   vi. Interprets treatment programme to the patients and concerned.
   vii. Facilitates continuity of the treatment when staff changes occur.
   viii. Facilitate in service training and student education program.
   ix. Evaluates effectiveness of the OT/PT intervention.
   x. Provides data for research and advancement of the professionals of OT/PT.

Do's and Dont's for Documentation in OT/PT

Do's

1. Be truthful, accurate and complete.
2. Write record as soon as treatment is rendered.
3. Date and sign all records.
4. Use specific terms.
5. Make factual statements.
6. Record broken appointments with reasons.
7. Record attempts to re-schedule.

Dont's

1. Change a record only after ascertaining the fact without clarifying when and why the change as made? What the nature of the change was?
2. Criticise another health care provider as part of the record.
3. Make judgmental statement about the patient and or his family.
4. Assume that the record will not be open to scrutiny by patient, family, lawyers and court.

Documentation abuse when it is

- Malpractice records
- Negligence and negligent recordings affect patient as: Loss to follow-up and reports
- Treatment record missing
- Side effects/implications of treatment effects. Patient does not comply with therapists instructions
- Diagnostic judgment was wrong
- Treatment outcomes bad even with best efforts put in
- Therapist faces a law suit.

Malpractice if

- Negligence in duty, poor standard of care, causes and damages to the health of patient.

Content and Process of Documentation in OT/PT

Record	Permanent record
Referral form data base	
Initial	
Data based evaluation	
Evaluation records	Summary
Treatment plan	Progress report
Running progress notes	Re-evaluation reports
Re-evaluation records	Progress report
Running progress notes	Discharge report

Functions of OT/PT

1. OT/PT is rehabilitating procedure guided by qualified professionals.
2. Need qualified prescription.
3. Uses various therapeutic means to cure.
4. Tries to gain physical and mental response.
5. Uses different modalities of treatment to make patients functionally viable.
6. Work in close relationship with other team members as desired/required.
7. Make patient return to the possible physical mental, social and economic independence.

Type of Records to be Maintained by Therapist

1. Keep records properly with agency also where employed with daily appointment records of patients for treatment.
2. Equipment purchase/repair/service records.
3. Keep patients financial records for audit in terms of
   a. Date of commencing treatment.
   b. Services obtained.
   c. Payments received by organization.
   d. Balance of account if any.

Document of Integrity of Records

- Accurately documenting records
- Policy (kind of records, time duration, true, accurate, complete records)
- Correct billing of treatment—Protect evidence for any chances of litigation.

Document Record Keeping Systems

It becomes more necessary for all of us so that proper and professional services are delivered for the satisfaction of the patient to keep records in computerized manner for preservation, referral and longevity.

Records are vital to process of management and monitoring of our services details to the patients.

They are useful if

- Provide evidence to support rule of law
- Support the accountability of work
- Are evidence of communication and discussions, actions, etc.
- Valuable in documenting trend, procedure and ways of management.

Type of Documents

i. Hand written on paper
ii. Typed on computer
iii. Records (files floppies, CDs, DVD VCD).

Documentation System

- Use integrated document system in institutional/organizational set-ups within the realities of the institute/organization
- Networking systems for number of personal computers being used in an organization help in transferring interdepartmental records
- Helps to strive to standardized and reduce paper work
- To give latest skills, procedures, management techniques, communication and support to keep record properly by the therapist.

Personnel Document

Classification of work force
- Full time
- Part time
- On wages.

Work position of therapist:
- Consultant
- Administrative
- Supervisor
- Staff therapist.

Work load policy document:
- General Policies
- Personnel considerations
- One therapist department
- Case load
- Designation of therapist.

Document of Business in Department

1. Filing of record:
   - Alphabetical and subject classification
   - Numerical classification
   - Alphabetical numerical classification.
2. Communications—Correspondence:
   - Telephone.
3. Budget.
4. Cost accounting.
5. Fees.
6. Purchasing.
   - Decentralize.
   - Controlled.
   - Centralized.
7. Equipment and supplies:
   - Classification.
   - Receipt and inventory.
   - Maintenance and repair.

Document Administrative Procedures

a. Safety procedure.
b. Emergency procedures:
   i. Fire safety.
   ii. Disaster program.
   iii. Other emergencies.
   iv. Disaster preparedness.

Document Treatment Procedures

a. Referral.
b. Treatment techniques.
c. Reporting and charting.
d. Attendance at OT/PT department.

Computerizing Patient Records

Computers have made a tremendous stride forward in preservation of the patient records, in medical science. Two important aspects in this behalf are.

1. Patients record keeping.
2. Printing of professional, prescription and reports including:
   a. Consent forms.
   b. Treatment notes.
   c. Evaluation reports.
   d. Progress reports.
   e. Discharge summary.
   f. Prescription cards.
   g. Health record proforma.
   h. Financial record proforma.
   i. Confidential record proforma.
   j. Legal heir record proforma.
   k. Emergencies as death/loss due to fire or theft.
   l. Protection against other person's mistakes or false statements, etc.

Document of Legal Aspects of Consumer Protection

Consumer Protection Act (CPA).

Document of Methods of Communication Policies, and Procedures

- Directive
- Manuals
- Specilty Memoranda, Bulletins, Newsletter
- Conference.

Reasons of Law Suit

1. Failure of monetary settlement.
2. For financial problems for patients.
3. Poor documenting of records.
4. Poor knowledge about disorders.
5. Fraudulent billing of treatment.
6. Well documented services minimize such suits.

Summary

During the past decade, record keeping has revolutionized in institutions and organizations. Now IT from mainframes to personal computers, to local area networks and internet has transformed the way agencies create, use, disseminate and store information.

These new technologies offer a vastly enhanced means of collecting information for and about patients, communication with state and people and agencies and document actions.

Many agencies have generated their computer records properly. Our concern over this ability is to preserve records properly for generations to refer in fulture. If you do not create record of your work, it is not excusable under law.

APPENDIX 3: COMPUTERIZATION OF DOCUMENTATION IN OCCUPATIONAL THERAPY

Occupational therapy also like any other profession has come to embrace the latest technological advances towards its development and sophistication as a science to treat and cure human beings.

Computerization has become an integral part of Occupational Therapy in treatment aspects, trainings aspects and in record, and preservation of the documents.

Wherever writing record is a part of service, it is observed that over a period of time, a good number of papers get accumulated in the files and to refer them in due course becomes an exercise. In recent past it has been observed that computers are well stablished as a mode of documenting and as a treatment tool in the all areas of OT.

Whilst the assessment and treatment applications are a well development schedule for documentation and research comparing computer use to more traditional methods is yet lacking.

The database yeilding the following profile of computer usage in OT neurology, elderly, general physical, mental handicap, psychiatry, orthopedics, pediatrics, young chronically sick is necessary.

While studying the extensive usage of computers in OT, some of the models in use in western world are in OT department as;

  i. BBC 'B', B + and masters 128.
 ii. PC and PC compatibles (Amstrad PC, OPUS, etc).
iii. Applied MAC and IIE (II comparable with BBC).
 iv. Amstrad PCW (dedicated work processor).
  v. Amiga 500.

The use of above models in OT for documentation and records of the therapy administration led to development of software and hardware for specific use of the OTs.

The BBC-Computers, in Special needs—education enabled the development of many switches, together with software, which OTs have been able to use with disabled people.

The full knowledge of hardware of computer system will be inclusive of microcomputer itself, monitor (Visual Display Unit), the disc drive and peripheral devices. Alternative input devices (Switches, concept Key boards) and output devices (Speech synthesisers) are also part of the hardware of system.

We need a basic package for OT departments consisting of microcomputer, color monitor, disk drive, printer, alternative inputs—joy sticks, concept, key board, touch screen (as per user's needs and necessity for objectives).

Slomo (Seven speed controller) or equivalent and suite of programs. There is need to ask few basic questions by the therapist for the most appropriate system. Some of the questions could be:

a. What is the computer required to do?
b. Is there sufficient power and memory in the computer?
c. How easy to connect the peripheral devices?
d. What kind of suitable software is available?

Input Device

Commonly used by OTs are:

- Concept—key board, touch screen
- Joy stick
- Mouse and tracker ball.

Types of Switches for Accessing Computer

- Double rocker switch
- Tilt switch
- Puff/suck switch
- Click switch
- Tongue switch
- Micro mike
- Head start (ultrasonic mouse emulator).

Inter Phase Box and Therapeutic Switches

- Inter phase box
- Slide switch
- large area pad switches

- Thumb switches
- Grip switch
- Double pull handle switch.

There are designated methods to put in the information into the computer by way of direct selection, scanning and encoded selection. The software has to be designed according to the needs of a particular OT department.

Modem is the device which can connect computer to telephone to have fast transfer of information from one computer to another to database and remote databases. Such systems make information accessible to disabled and nondisabled persons.

The various program suites can be of:

a. Perception
b. Motor ability
c. Congnition
d. Life skills—ADL
e. Work skills
f. Education types.

In addition, we need to do software evaluation in terms of the level of the program, its age appropriateness, points to look in for design and content, whether documentation is available and what kind of hardware and peripherals are required to run it. Such evaluation criteria needs to be drawn for the befitting documentation of OT service.

While developing a software keep points as under in mind:

- Knowing what you want to do
- Knowing how to do it efficiently and effectively
- Evaluating whether it has been done correctly or not. Three fold assessment of the developed software is to be made in terms of
  - Quality of the program
  - Function of the program
  - Effect of the program in treatment setting.

Copyrights of the softwares should be respected totally.

- Computers have therapeutic application in OT as under to which Data Protection Act (1984) is applicable.

- Physical dysfunction:
    - Locomotor dysfunction
    - Sensory impairment.
- Neurological dysfunction:
    - Physical problems
    - Cognitive problems
    - Perceptual problems.
- Life skills; such as ADL:
    - Self care
    - Work
    - Lesisure
    - Social skills
    - Communication
    - Education.

Psychological Consideration

Many persons have fear to use these computers psychologically. It can be overcome by first using switches of any electronic gadget of day-to-day use.

Computers make strong motivational considerations. User friendly software should be used for making it a consistently usable without fear and anxiety.

Use of computers in OT department of the institutions/centers/hospitals is the basis of budget and motivation to upgrade service delivery with sophisticated methods with more care and skill requirements.

The attitudes to promote sophistication in therapy services is at present neglected area except at certain places.

I strongly advocate that since occupational therapy is the highly vital component of health giving system, all practising OTs should equip themselves with the latest technological advances to be fully embraced with services quality they are delivering. She should have a combination of traditional therapy modes and new advances incorporated to make her therapy more effective and efficient.

APPENDIX 4: ROLE OF OCCUPATIONAL THERAPY PREVENTING INDOOR POLLUTION

Pollution is a greatest threat ever to human life which needs to be attended to by the community of the occupational therapists of our country. We can understand Pollution in two types, i.e. indoor and outdoor. The outdoor pollution gets neutralized to an extent that it may be diluted to affect human body but it is not always so. The serious threat is posed by indoor air pollution to which many of the human beings of various ages are exposed to most of their life-spans.

The indoor pollution is generally in homes, schools, offices. Picture halls, under one roof markets, shopping malls, hospitals, community centers, etc. with this we see that health professionals are thrown challenge under such circumstances. The individuals who are presenting with environmentally associated symptoms are opting to have been exposed to airborne substances originating not outdoors, but indoors.

The industrialized nations spend 90 percent of their time indoors. For children, aged, disabled with chronic diseases, most of the events where such problems occur. Three problems need careful examination of the pollutants as in case of allergies, influenza and common cold. Many effects may be associated with stress, work pressure and seasonal discomforts.

Some of the noticeable indoor air pollution may be environmental tobacco smoke and sick building syndrome need to be brought to notice of public attention and suggestions of connection between respiratory or other symptoms in home or workplace of which we need to make the individuals of such places and produce awareness.

The mild symptoms can be cared for and may be avoided with precautions/prevention measures for healthy living workplaces. The signs and symptoms in infants and children are atypical. A chart can be drawn in the form of strains can be taken care of by occupational therapy role many folds.

Occupational Therapists can investigate by matching the individuals signs and symptoms to those pollutants category for which, the checklist of OT can be somewhat on these lines as under:

1. When did symptoms occur or complaint made?
2. Does it exist all the time or not?
3. Are you in the same place when symptoms occur?
4. Does the problem cease immediately or gradually?
5. What is your work?
6. Have you changed your employer or assignments?
7. Has employer changed location of your work or not?
8. Has place been redecorated or refurnished?
9. Have you started working with new or different materials?
10. What is the smoking policy at your work place?
11. Are you exposed to environmental tobacco smoke at work, school, home, etc.?
12. Describe your work area.
13. Have you recently changed your place of residence?
14. Have made any changes recently in your home, office, etc. or additions?
15. Have you recently acquired a new pet?
16. Does any one else in your home have similar problems? Or any one with whom you work?(if yes it may be common source or a communicable disease).

In addition to above, occupational therapist can play a vital role in prevention of indoor air pollution by addressing to above questions. Environmental tobacco smoke (ETS) is major source of indoorair containment. ETS in indoor air environment indicate that some unintentional inhalation of ETS by non-smokers is unavoidable. ETS is a dynamic, complex mixture of more than 4,000 chemicals found in both vapors and particle phases. Many chemicals out of these are carcinogenic substances which will occur in indoor space where there is smoking. This warrants a major attention by OTs to make public awareness of these facts to prevent such health threats in masses. The remedial action by occupational therapists can be:

a. Improve general ventilation in indoor spaces in the above listed places.
b. Whenever generally accepted ventilation methods fail, there by word of mouth through camps and public education, the intentions are achieved.

c. In the instances of complex gaseous mixtures and particulate components the general ventilation measures do not work. Provide separately designed smoking rooms for the smokers for the purpose if very essential.

d. Use of higher efficiency air cleaning systems, under some select conditions can be installed.

e. Air cleaners (desk top model) of the same may not be effective. Even some are designed but are not effective to remove dangerous gases.

f. Tobacco control is a must and it is essential to invest more time in eradication through campaigns of educating public on health hazards of these consumables to human life.

g. Most affected are children and their lungs are more vulnerable due to poor body resistance build in system.

Remedial Action by OTs

i. Provide adequate outdoor air ventilation to dilute human source aerosols.

ii. Keep equipment water reservoirs clean and potable water systems adequately chlorinated as per manufacturers instructions.

iii. See that there is no stagnant water in air conditioners.

iv. Repair leaks and seepages.

v. Thoroughly clean and dry water damaged carpets, any building materials within 24 hrs of damage or remove or replace.

vi. Keep relative humidity below 50 percent.

vii. Use exhaust fans in bathroom, kitchen and vent clothes dryers to outside.

viii. Control exposure to pets.

ix. Use vaccum cleaners for carpets and upholstery of furniture.

x. Keep areas dust free as much as possible.

xi. Cleaning, re-suspends fine particles during and immediately after the activity.

xii. Sensitive individuals to be cautioned of dusty/polluted environments, etc.

xiii. Use commercially available HEPA (high efficiency particulate air) filtered vaccum.

xiv. Cover mattresses.

xv. Wash bedding and soft toys frequently in water at a temperature above 130°F to kill dust mites.

Biological air pollutants are found in every home, school and workplace. Sources are outdoor aid of human occupants who shed viruses and bacteria, animals occupants, i.e. insects and other arthropods, mammals, etc. that shed allergens and indoor surfaces and water reservoirs where fungi and bacteria, grow such as humidifiers are important to be taken cognizance of factors which allow biological agents to grow release into air are:

a. High humidity increases dust mite population in house in damp places so avoid it.

b. Mite and fungus contamination by flooding, damp carpets on poor damp flooring—so avoid it.

c. Mechanical heating, ventilating and air conditioning systems may cause to serve as reservoirs of microbial amplification so may be avoided.

The biological agents in indoor air cause three types of human disease: Injections where pathogens invade human tissues:

• Hypersensitivity diseases causing specific activation of the immune system causes disease

• Toxicosis where biologically produced chemical toxin cause direct toxic effects.

Biological contaminations, i.e. dampness of water damage are related to non-specific upper and lower respiratory symptoms, sick building syndrome is related to microbial contamination in buildings as discussed earlier.

Occupational therapists are the community contact persons directly and hence are most apt to perform preventive education role to masses on the hazards and management ways of the indoor-air contamination pollution.

APPENDIX 5: OCCUPATIONAL THERAPY WHILE UPDATING

It is inevitable that any professional has to update his knowledge as per time requirements. No education remains stand still. The knowledge bank in human brain grows day and night as the professional grows.

What is the essential ingredient of growth of any knowledge? Nothing else but updating the latest what ever is the development taking place.

Occupational therapy has traversed a considerable path in this part of the world and has found a suitable place inservice delivery systems of rehabilitation of the physically handicapped/mentally subnormals or retarded and psychiatric cases. In the last few years the area of drug abuse has also been invaded by occupational therapy thereby giving a more dimention to its earlier facets of dimentions.

In present times its application in hospitals, rehabilitation centers, nursing homes, private clinics of various medical men is seen. OTs are also running their own private clinics. When these practice areas are critically analyzed, one feels clearly that private practice and institutional attachment models show the use of this methodology in the area of physical disability. Secondly, it is also observed that practice in private clinic models in the area of psychiatry and mental retardation is nil. This practice model is limited to certain institutional models only. As is also evident for the practice in drug abuse. The OT as such has not been explotied by each qualified OT in herself/ himself so far. Perhaps due to this, we land up into crisis of identity with physical therapists because of this reason only.

More areas which can be tapped in addition to above, various models are:

i. **Preventive Practice Model of OTs:** Where the OTs can find attachments with big industrial set ups to advise the employers to observe safety measures for workers at working situations to avoid paying compensations to injured later on.

ii. **Functional Training Practice Model:** This could be both for institutional and noninstitutional model cases where actual ADL training is carried out in the live situations of the cases as the need may call for.

iii. **Mobile-Live Training Model Practice:** This means that the services of an OT could be hired by a prospective case who can afford to pay a salary to a therapist and keeps him or her with himself all through his day's regime of work. This helps both OT to get a live difficulty situation of the patient and provide a solution then and there only and the patient gets on the spot attention when he is in difficulty to excute a certain action.

This practice model has been started very recently in Delhi as the patient could afford a handsome salary to attached OT with him from 10.00 AM to 8.00 PM daily.

iv. **Forensic Practice Model:** This model is not available yet in our country. This needs to be developed and there is everybody's concern in that spirit. The legal practice model will be very beneficial in the industrial set-ups in our country because industrialization in our country with sophistication of equipments has made it imparative to think on this model of practice of this profession also.

The factors prompting the changes in the practice models in its widening base are as:

- Social changes
- Changing health care scene
- OT employment trends
- OT practice trends
- Emerging career options
- Tomorrow's health care
- Potential changes in OT practice
- Potential changes in education
- Potential changes in research
- Directions for the future
- Maintaining traditional values in a changing society. Like this we find that the science of occupation to help the human capacities is a fruitful gain of OT professionals who strive to cure or alleviate the inabilities of their cases in day-to-day life.

APPENDIX 6: ACCESS TO RURAL ENVIRONMENT

Access is reach and I feel when we have thought of it, we have reached the villages where our most of the population is dwelling under the most natural settings of the life. They breath fresh air than the urban population who is breathing air with smoke and dust of the vehicles and of the towering chimneys of the power houses and dust around.

It is felt that the urbanization of the village's may be a step to disturb the peace prevailing there but grooming strides of the technology make it essential that these steps taken forwards must be utilized in improvization of the rural setups. It is also seen and observed that day-to-day activities and various others chores of the people are such; which do not pose grave problems to the experts of any field.

When we talk of the rehabilitation services being made available to the handicapped in the cities we mean that must also be made available to those who are living in villages where their parents have already settled through generations. Bringing the villager to a city in a hospital/rehabilitation center for any type of training depending upon his/her nature of the handicap shall not solve our purpose of his rehabilitation. His resettlement into his way of life, before getting handicapped to achieve this, we require to have a close observation of the type of job, position of the concerned in performing his work, position and posture requirements of the work. All these shall determine, the extent up to which the rehabilitation services are required in his case. Like this we get various examples which shall need a close observation. These observation can only be possible when a rehabilitation expert has full orientation to rural setups and ways of life of the rural people so that he can do his best to rehabilitate the concerned to his maximum.

Many persons feel and think that rehabilitation experts in urban life can do full justice to rehabilitate the villagers with various types of handicaps but it is not absolutely correct. The experts diverted to the rural population must be oriented fully about the circumstances prevailing and nature of the lifestyle of the people in villages so that while prescribing or describing any type of job to the handicapped person, may helps solve the problems of the later.

What at present we find that a rehabilitation team, is sent for a visit to a village which is adopted and surveyed. These members of the team are the parsons who have never lived in a village and hence cannot appraise themselves of the problems of the villagers completely though the villagers may express in their regional language which may or may not be understood fully by the team. It is not always the procedure to depute the regional person who knows the local language fully so that the language barrier is overcome up to some extent in the measures taken to rehabilitate the handicapped.

It is therefore, suggested that the various types of training centers, ITI, and workshops be setup in the villages so that the handicapped villagers may not have to walk/travel a long distance to reach the training center and face the accommodation and conveyance problems which can easily be solved by providing the centers for rehabilitation and training of the handicapped in their respective places of their residence or with hostel facilities for the period of training as specified for particular job/trade.

The various types of the training jobs should be such that they are rural oriented jobs which are mostly performed by the uneducated and educated villagers. For example, farming, poultry raising, pig raising, small industry, weaving and various other such occupations. The center so designed for the purpose shall try to fulfill the needs of that particular village population. The essential requirements can be met easily by the center. The requirements of food, grinding masalas, making of shoes/chappals, weaving cloth-coarse and fine, pottery, etc. can be few suggested jobs. Then in due course a departmental store can he raised with low construction cost from where every villager can buy the articles of his utility. The wealth so earned by the village may be used in the same village to develop the center and expand its activities. When the products go surplus they may be brought to cities and sold there. I will like to add here that handloom cloth has become a craze of the day, as it provides a wide range of color, design and quality both in cotton and silk. Like this, the various other items of perfection can be introduced both in villages and cities. Very recently, the match boxes fancy ones, have come into the markets from Khadi and Village Industries. It is seen that these products which are already in the markets from the villages are in no way inferior to those from cities.

I very emphatically add that India's wealth is in the villages. The villages are the treasures which are very valuable and precious to the country and hence must be made use of fully in the betterment of the nation.

Now, take the other aspect to access the provision of the gadgets to the handicapped of the villages. The gadgets should be simple to use and in design, low cost and not cumbersome so that they may be used without any difficulty. And due to the repeated use, it require minor repairs and adjustments which can be done by the wearer himself. If the center is not in his village then a repair of say ₹ 5/- shall become exorbitant when he has to travel miles by train and then may have to stay in a rented accommodation and needs to spend for food as well, which when calculated may cost roughly ₹ 200/- or so. He may think all that, postpone the idea of repair of the gadget and shall deteriorate his condition without a gadget further. If an artificial limb is provided to a farmer, it should be kept in mind that the limb should be so sturdy and strong which can bear the strain of this body weight when he is working whole day in the feld marshy muddy farm. The raw material used should be washable so that the mud, etc. can be cleaned with water and the limb dried with cloth later on.

Similarly, the caliper and the short leg braces should be strong which do not give way soon. This can be checked and maintained by choosing a simple design of manufacture.

The sticks with strong rubber tips and crutches with good strength may also be advised to be used as they will not break soon.

The wheelchairs should not be of metal and with sophisticated adjustments because the simple mind of the villagers may not be in a position to achieve speed and efficiency in operation; so therefore, the wheel chairs may be of teak wood with wooden strong wheel which may be painted with a waterproof paint. The design may be so simple of the wheelchair can be manufactured in the rehabilitation center of the village only.

The recommendations for a rehabilitation center can only be successful when, where the center is to be opened should have a large number of the various categories of the handicapped to make it multi category or otherwise as the case may be. The local village authorities may approach the government for the financial assistance or banks who give loans on low rates of interests for small scale industry and rehabilitation centers to be setup. Like this we, find that the multi-angular approach is to be made in such ventures so that the publicity of the work is also maintained and the considerable encouragement is met from the public at large. The various voluntary agencies for the welfare of the handicapped should join hands with the government at all ranks and files 'to propagate the cause of the handicapped from city to city and village to village to make the efforts a glorious success in as a manner as possible at all costs so that the rehabilitation catches momentum with dynamic, force behind.

APPENDIX 7: OCCUPATIONAL THERAPY: MAKING NEEDED CHANGES

The transformation in thinking and problem-solving is a long standing and familiar orientation to occupational therapists. As early as 1910, OT embraced the recognition that an individual health was bound up in the intricacies of daily experience in a complex and social world. This science got organized around the concept of occupation and profession has from its beginning, using notions of self satisfaction in daily living, balance in work, play, sleep and rest, mastery and competence, learning through activity and practice for real life situations—as the underpinnings of treatment.

Disease and disability have always been viewed as disruptions in a person's life and the goal of intervention has always been to reestablish habits and skills that would insure a personal return to a satisfying life. This has always been the concern of occupational therapists.

In 1980s and beyond, survival of OT is not dependent, on our ability to change our way of thinking from mechanistic systems view. We have always treated the whole person. The treatment procedures and plans are based on factors like interest, values, goals into the plans of the treatment.

In a sense, more than ever OT is an idea whose time has come. The long standing professional expertise that we all possess in occupation and associated areas that include recognition of the importance of survival skills, the relationship between curiosity and activity are the basis for inter vention strategies that insure an individuals adaptation to the environment.

Our survival as a profession depends more on our ability to act quickly and effectively in response to the changing needs and environments in health care.

The service occupational therapists provide is vital today and will be in even greater demand in the tomorrows of this decades. The greatest challenge to occupational therapy lies in our ability to communicate what we do and how our service will benefit people, their family and society.

Role of Occupational Therapist

When ADL treatment medium has advanced rapidly and has made great progress in use and acceptance, it is still a field in which participation open to many interested persons. Not only doctors, occupational therapists, physiotherapists, nurses and patients themselves may become involved but orthotists and special technicians have been added to the team in many places. Interested volunteers and manufacturers have made many contributions and today more and more designers and engineers are devoting their skills to help to solve the problems.

Occupational therapists today may participate on many levels. With their skills in the use of tools and materials, their knowledge and understanding of various physical disabilities and physical function because they have the facilities of workshop available. Frequently they may be called on to fabricate devices even if only temporary ones. Because of their interest in this field many occupational therapists have already made outstanding contributions, today, because of the increasing supply of commercial devices. The gradual interest in the training of orthotists, the need for occupational therapist to make devices themselves is lessening gradually. However, in the role of evaluation of devices including testing and training the occupational therapist is and probably always will be key performer. Although he/she should continue to give assistance whenever needed, according to development in his/her locality or institution, the main emphasis of the role described here will be laid upon testing and training.

Psychological Aspects

This aspect is of special importance and is of consideration of psychological reaction of the patient in relation to the use of mechanical aids or devices. Some of the factors found to influence their satisfactory acceptance and use are:

i. *Interest:* May be influenced by any of the other reactions or by the patients feeling that he is sick and can not depending on the duration and extent of the disability.

ii. *Age:* May be a liability or an asset or may not be important.

iii. *Reaction to the new and different:* Some persons are inspired by new ideas. The majority tends to favor accustomed and previously accepted methods of doing things.

iv. *Cosmetic factors:* One of the goals of the rehabilitation is to give the greatest possible appearance of normalcy whenever it can be done.

v. *Social cultural factors:* Feeling of the acceptance by the society, at home or in some social gathering.

The Devices

Before prescribing any type of device, assistive of course, we have to keep many points in our mind which will lead to successful acceptance by the patient and purpose for which it is designed. The various points to be considered are:

i. *Mechanical aspects:* The design or fabrication of a device may not be the responsibility of the occupational therapists. However, even if it is not, knowledge of essential factors enhances his own understanding of devices fabricated by others or of those available commercially. This does not men that the occupational therapists should be expected to add all the skills of mechanical engineering to his own present training or that he uses only of his acquired bits of knowledge to infringe on the responsibilities of the other team members. It is suggested only that if he makes devices he should be equipped with as much know-how as possible.

If he participates only in testing and their method of fabrication is invaluable in getting expectation of performance of device itself and in knowing where to look for true trouble spots.

ii. *Time:* Patient's need marks time for the construction. If the patient's interest is ilicited try to supply the devices as quickly as possible. Waiting decreases his receptiveness. But beware of poor construction and unsuitable materials which reduce durability in case of operation. Break downs are frustrating also.

iii. *Materials:* Select the material according to the patients needs. Weighing factors like, weights, strength, flexibility, durability, washability, life expectancy and color against cost and method of fabrication and facilities for construction. Most of the new plastics and many metals can be handled successfully in a small shop with a minimum amount of experience.

iv. *Construction:* The key note is simplification and durability. The less complicated the construction, the more quickly and easily can one meet the demand. Durability results in fewer repairs and visits to the workshops. Both these needs are best answered through better knowledge of materials.

v. *Operation:* This factor of necessity go hand in hand with the construction. Usually simplication of construction means ease of use. However, this may not be true in regard to sliding parts, where friction may have to be eliminated. And here, we must refer again to the individual needs of the patients disability, intellectual functioning, manual dexterity and the environment.

vi. *Design:* Depends upon all other factors plus the cosmetic needs. Good design usually has its foundation, the basic principles of good construction. Modern architecture offers many fine examples. Beauty of construction and function can go hand in hand.

vii. *Manufacturing aspects*
   a. Extent and/or amount of use.
   b. Availability and cost of the materials.
   c. Interpretation of requirement of the devices for the production.
   d. Construction details.
   e. Operation or how to use it.
   f. Manufacturing goals.
   g. Estimate of potential market and distribution.

viii. *Training:* Just as a person cannot be expected to drive a car properly without learning or to perform an acrobatic feast with excellence without repeated practice, so a person with a new device may need a period of training in its use. Never should a patient be discharged without the opportunity first to perform successfully whatever activity is undertaken. There are some cardinal rules:

a. Learning something may take a long time. It is a process, not a end result, so allow adequate time for practice.

b. Mistakes are a part of learning. If not repeated too often, they may even be helpful. They may remind us of precautions and may suggest that there may be better ways.

c. The patient may have valuable suggestions to offer. Listen carefully and objectively before rejecting ideas different from your own.

d. Keep alert to better and more effective methods of training. Enthusiasm properly controlled is always an essential.

e. Even though careful planning has been given to designing a device in actual use, one may find that certain adjustments or modifications are necessity.

Therefore, it is the occupational therapist, who is the whole sole designer of these assistive devices which will solve all the problems involving disorganization of activities of daily living. They are the architects of the hopes of these diabled, a community of invalids.

APPENDIX 8: OCCUPATIONAL THERAPY AND ENVIRONMENT

There is a saying that a healthy mind in a healthy body but to achieve this we need to create an environment for the same.

It is therefore very necessary to understand what an environment is surrounding, a team of persons around OT in any setting, housing an individual in four walls of the community setting, a disabled at home, work place and public place.

With this vast domain of understanding environment for an OT it is very clear to understand the vast applications of this versatile science of human skills in extraordinary manner.

The presentation discusses certain aspects which need care and attention of occupational therapist working in departmental setting or in private practice model.

In addition to certain other aspects we can consider forensic occupational therapist which deals with legal aspects of the practice in industrial setup. This area at present in India hardly finds any place. No occupational therapist even has ever tried to venture his/her skills in this aspect of practice. The rate of industrial accidents has proportionately increased in past few years. All such injured workers are in the dilemma of being shunted out of employment or those who have been compensated they are not satisfied as to be just ready to work elsewhere or come up in self-employment.

While considering the expansion of OT environment, one thinks of the areas to work in:

    I. Dress designing for the disabled.

    II. Active domiciliary model of OT in our country.

    III. Mobile services model.

The areas of dress designing need an active initative by OT because many disabled temporarly or permanently are not in a position to dress up properly or cannot do so. It is therefore, becomes essential area where speciality is achieved to facilitate the dressing-up by the patients themselves who cannot or find it difficult to do so.

This will need an indepth examination and evaluation of ADL extensively with special detailed evaluation on dressing abilities.

It has been observed that the disabled when discharged, in number of cases, do not possess ADL independence in total. Some how, in some cases, the treatment falls short of the man hour session on extensive functional independence training to disabled.

In the hospital setups, it is seen that ADL training finds hardly any place in hospital model working. If at all this exists, it is for this, as a whole. The team of such training may consist of
- Medical specialist, medical social worker
- Occupational therapist (active member)
- One or two attendants as the case may be
- Nurse to assist in total procedure.

There is need and its an essential component of total rehabilitation of any permanently disabled case. It can be for short lived difficulties in ADL also.

In addition to above, the work situation environment should also be improved. In many instance it has come to notice that the staff of OT department is not having congenial relationship among themselves thns work environement becomes sick. It not only reflects on its functioning but also causes lot of difficulty in administration of department and service alongwith defective documentation.

The work environment is dependent on:
  i. Attitude
  ii. Sincerity
  iii. Type of work
  iv. Consistency in work
  v. Willingness to work
  vi. Work spirit.

In general there are other work constraints like less flow of funds.
- Inadequate equipment
- Lack of space
- Nonavailability of required number of staff in the department.

Like this, we see that environment is a very big and broad term which cannot be afforded to be misunderstood in limited sense. A healthy service can be provided from occupational therapist only when a keen environment exists.

APPENDIX 9: ATTITUDES IN PROVISION OF THE FUNCTIONAL AIDS AND APPLIANCES TO THE HANDICAPPED

Functional aids and appliances are used when other rehabilitative measures do not bear fruits. It may also be understood in other words as perhaps the professionals do not have patience and time to exhaust various procedures to achieve a particular function but to advice these aids and appliances.

In many instances, the patients themselves are in a hurry and exhibit their eagerness to be functional in the shortest span possible. In certain cases, it becomes very difficult to curb such tendencies in patients. This sometimes caused inadequate approach in acceptance of appliance/aid or its usefulness on its functional utility. Such hurries should be avoided to experience failures by patient or by the provider.

The functional ability promoted helps to creat independence in day-to-day tasks and functions which one needs to perform.

The application of aids will be determined by the competence achieved by the patient who is using it. How sturdy it is, how often it needs repairs? What kind of repairs? Can it be handled by the user himself or needs to be taken for repairs? In later case, it can take long-time which hampers individual's routine a bit so the user gets upset and develops sometime a no use attitude. It is therefore, suggested that the design, material, etc. should be such which leads to break downs to the minimum possible. The attitude of the manufacturer or designer should be on its easy use and maximum utility without difficulty.

The appliances and aids should be cosmetically good. It is often rejected by the patient on the plea that it is not of good appearance. Like this, patient does not get motivated frequently and often use it for performance. Many such appliances laid become a wasteful expenditure rather than otherwise.

The fabrication, design, mechanism, cosmesis are important factors club together to make it a "NO REJECT" by the patients. In addition to this, the factor of fatigue also play a role. It should be mechanically sound that undue stresses and strains are not caused to produce discomfort in the wearer or the user.

Another area to be affected by the attitudes is the proper training to the user. Due to increasing incidence of the disability, the quality service has been greatly affected because there has not been corresponding proportional increase of man power needed.

When there is full devotion by the therapist in the work, the patient cannot escape from their due right of getting fully rehabilitated. The attitudes are greatly influenced by the consistency, zeal and spirit of working. This matters a lot in the welfare services for the diabled. The working with handicapped is in itself an attitude thus the service is closely affected by its decrease or increase. These attitudes are reflected in fittings of the aids and appliance by the professionals.

The use of computer for alignment checks and for other reasons can be extensively placed at the service of the professional. Alignment factor is also very important while considering attitudinal factors.

The use and provision of the aids and appliances is as essential as any thing else to handicapped. The acceptance is shown with full use and utility of the item by the concerned diabled. It is seen that the disabled who accept it, use it fully and accept as part of their self.

The extra devotion of time to the training of the disabled with aids and appliances is keyword for its successfulness in its total functions and freedom.

Activities of Daily Living Interpretation and Assistive Devices

The uniform application and interpretation of the activities of daily living is more difficult than that of the muscle test since the ADL test is a performance test of gross musculoskeletal selected movement. The benefits of uniform application and the interpretation, however, cannot be achieved until the methods for activities of daily living are standardized. The first step towards this has been materialized with the publication of Edith Buchwald's Physical rehabilitation for Daily Living in 1952.

The achievement of functional independence in the performance of those activities which must be accomplished each day in order to enable a person to live at home and participate in modern society is one of the goals of rehabilitation. These activities are known as activities of daily living or self-care.

In course of everyday life each person must perform or be assisted in performing such activities as:

a. Arising from bed
b. Caring for hygiene
c. Eating
d. Dressing
e. Using the wheelchairs
f. Ambulating and performing a wide variety of manual tasks.

Any person who cannot accomplish all these activities will be dependent on others for help everyday.

Though patient may have great deal of useful physical abilities the inability to perform one or more of the essential activities of daily living leaves him dependent on others.

Degree of Independence

The goal of each ADL program is to train the patient for maximum independence in carrying out his daily activities. According to their specific ability to move effectively patients attain different degrees of independence.

Though, the goal is independence in the wheelchair as well as in activities requiring ambulation, this is not always possible or practical. The actual goals are measured by

a. Extent of disability
b. Age
c. Occupation
d. Home
e. Work situation which are influenced by the factors as:
   • Some are exceptional patients who are completely dependent on an assistant but still incharge of their business

- The functional indepence does not depend on ability to walk in ones day-to-day life. Many wheelchair bounds are certainly able to work and hold a job if can perform the activities like.
  - Bed activities including transfers in bed
  - Wheelchair activities and transferes
  - Self-care activities
  - Driving a car—with hand controls.

Standard of Performance

As soon as ADL program is determined consisting of set of activities for evaluation necessiates to define standard performance terms of evaluation to understand our own version what we say. It is often seen that no body understands what one is talking about.

While analyzing the patients skills and abilities on activities he either can do or cannot do with or without help. The necessary kind of help may be in terms of:

- lifting the patient
- The entire activity being done for the patient
- Patient needing assistance
- Patient supervision.

What Do We Mean by Independence?

If a patient can carry out a given activity entirely by himself with required amount of speed and endurance with assistance or otherwise means he is functionally independent. The patient may repeat the activity number of times in a day without getting tired or exhausted.

The Use of Devices

We do find in our daily life that devices, i.e. assistive devices become inevitable in certain disability handicap and also in many chronic disabilities where no functional return full or partial is visible without device. These devices though assist the patient to perform certain functions successfully are the only way to succeed with these functionally difficult cases.

The application of the assistive devices poses challenges to the practicing occupational therapists. Each disabled individual will face a different approach of an occupational therapist during his training towards fuller functional rehabilitation in certain cases of the disabled.

Thus, I very strongly feel here that we all face an open challenge to plan and device simple, low cost, easy to make, easy to manoeuver self-help and assistive devices. The complicated technology keeps the patient in a very difficult situation where he fails to operate the said assistive device or is so heavy that does not choose to either use or wear the same. You may realise that his choice to do so is at the cost of his functional excellence in his day-to-day performance of daily tasks.

The ADL training with or without assistive devices is very useful part of total training required for the rehabilitation of the handicapped.

Maintenance of hygiene: The usual hygenic activities of washing brushing teeth, brushing hair, shaving or applying make-up, combing hair and using a handkerchief may require assistive device to make each of the function listed above easy. Limitation to learn mobility or of grasp interfere with the performance of these activities.

Training program: While concentrating on the training of daily activities we have to simultaneously also use other therapies to improve muscle power wherever possible, coordination and range of movement if restricted. The proper head and trunk control in neurological deficits are the basic ingredients to properly coordinate the purposeful movement with or without assistive devices for proper ADL training program.

The use of the assistive devices is essential to achieve the therapy objectives towards functional freedom of any disabled person.

Therefore, evaluation of improvement in self-care becomes meaningful only when effective comparison can be made of patients abilities before and after rehabilitation.

Some of the patients fall under the groups of disability which can be helped in effective activities training program with few standard assistive devices where as others require both thought and time to device for the handicapped individual.

Psychological reactions and motives: They are varied in individual case and are accordingly to be attend to. The common psychological problem being faced by practicing occupational therapists is that of non cooperation of many of the disabled patients while training them in ADL with or without devices as, for example, in strokes.

This disrespect of the disability in the mind of the disabled is one of the major factors to produce such reactions in their minds. The disease though is to prolong but it is not accepted by the disabled himself causing mental unrest.

Whereas such problems are not very much evident in developmentaly handicapped individuals. Therefore, it is very necessary to take full account of these difficulties also while training the disabled in activities of daily living.

Extent/jurisdiction of ADL training: There is actually no limit to such a training. It will solely depend upon the type of job he was involved in and life style of that particular disabled person. The procedure, style and type of training desired in particular case shall be determined only after detailed functional assessment of the individual case.

While making such an evaluation, we have also to consider the types of the self-help devices being used by the patient, if so which were provided inorder to enable him perform any particular activity successfully which otherwise was not possible.

ADL training shall be considerd incomplete without the use of the assistive devices which make the disabled functionally independent. This training tries to provide freedom to the patient to function independently at home or outside, i.e. at his office, shop or elsewhere.

I would very much appreciate here if treating occupational therapist can also make home/work/shop visits so as to actually visualise the various problems being encountered by that disabled person accordingly.

Many patients maintain a high degree of function despite limitation or deformities in fingers, wrists and shoulders. Heavy work is often very difficult or impossible. Often the delicate or precision work, but activities of daily living, house hold work and many forms of gainful employment are maintained if the disease permits.

When joint limitations impairs essential functions, the need of appropriate self-help devices arises. Such consideration would have to be accounted for in the self-care activities for the patients.

While concluding it can be said that training in activities of daily living and use of assistive devices is very essential to achieve functional freedom in the disabled.

APPENDIX 10: ACCESS PROVISIONS FOR THE DISABLED CHILDREN IN THE SCHOOLS

Access means way to or into a place. The children need very easy access approaches in the surroundings which enable them to learn and grow both physically and mentally. So is the case with disabled children also. It is more necessary and needed in later case because their disability may hamper their free movement with or without aids affecting their accessibility in places like schools.

The access considerations are in case of the physically handicapped and sometimes for other disabilities also where ever their functional freedom is at stake. Generally, the access provisions are considered at home, place of work, public places and conveniences, etc.

The access provisions in schools will be in:

a. *Staircases:* The staircases can be provided with side railing at reasonable level from each step above 18 to 20 inches. These fixtures should be very strong to bear the downward force being exerted by the child. The height of these additional support railing will be different for different age group children on an average growth standards.

   The steps should be a wide and about 9 inches wide and about 8 inches high so that there is easy lifting of the foot to 8 inches height. Width of 9 inches is sufficient to provide stability base of the foot. While alternating the foot in assending or descending the staircase.

b. *Classroom:* The classrooms as far as possible may be on the ground floor only with special considerations to disabled child class. If the architecture of the school building does not permit easy access for the child/children, then above measure only is the answer.

   In case, school funds permit provisions then required alterations in the classroom can be provided like: special classroom with adapted furniture for individual disabled child's requirement.

The width of doors leading to classrooms must be adequate. It may be 3 to 3.5 feet if possible for the conventient wheelchair movements in and out of classroom. It is essential for wheelchair movements.

c. *Toilets:* Same we need to observe for doors for toilets also as for classroom doors. More so, the inside room of toilet should be minimum 6 × 6 feet with toilet seats facing door of the toilet as far as possible.

In already constructed toilets, the wheel chair maneuvering may be bit difficult for school children of any age. Children of smaller age group of school may have a smaller model of wheel chairs and adult model for adult groups of school children.

d. *Library:* Generally, the school should have library facilities little away from classrooms on ground level only. It may be there in many schools in basement or at any floor of the building as suitably decided by that school administration.

Therefore, it is same for doors to be of the size of classrooms, toilets, etc. or doors any where in school premises which can allow wheelchairs, if any, of disabled.

e. *Assembly hall:* As far as should be on ground level. If not then either ramps may also be provided along with stairs or whole of the school building should have lifts incase some children are wheelchair bound. Those with calipers and crutches or sticks would need for training for which local near by institutions for disabled be tapped or 1 pH may be tapped.

f. *Canteen:* Tables and chairs in the canteen should be of the height which children can use comfortably. If not on ground floor, children may have an easy access to canteen through ramp, stairs or lift as the case may be.

For doors, etc. the size has to be minimum 3.5 to 4 feet for easy movement of the wheelchairs. There may be railing provision along the walks of the canteen, classroom, library, toilets, bathroom, common room, recreation rooms and all the corridors and stair cases invariably for barest possible access provision with an attitude from the each school principal to accommodate each disabled pupil also in school to promote integrated educational policy of government by providing facilities for the disabled and normal children alike under one roof.

ANNEXURE 11: OCCUPATION THERAPY IN HAND INJURIES

Introduction

Hand can work miracles in the world of today in the fields of science, technology, medicine and rehabilitation. The machine age—modern times has made hand a victim of various kinds of the injuries involving, muscles, joints, tendons, tissues and nerves in a part of a body or parts of the body. They may also get amputated partly or fully.

The chemicals handling, electrical short circuits, mishandling of electrical goods, etc. can also injure hands in minor or major form resulting into a disability—temporary or permanent with or without complications.

The thermal burns may produce injuries which render hand function less partially or totally.

The therapy planned for the hand aims at the full successful use of the hand though with partial or full return of its functions. Therefore, the need of the splints also arises during or after the treatment of the hand abnormalities.

Many a times, the recovery of the function in hand abnormalities is fully dependent on the effective planning of occupational therapy for which detailed knowledge of the hand functions is a must for the occupational therapist who is handling the case.

Functions of the Hand

The human hand has three primary functions; it is an organ of investigation, a grasping mechanism and an instrument of expression.

The Power Grip

This is a function of the long flexor tendons to which thenar and hypothenar muscles add the ability to close the palm around an object and other intrinsic muscles contribute a stabilizing influence. For this, crude, protective sensation is sufficient.

The Precision Grip

This is a balanced action between the extrinsic and the intrinsic muscles, in which thumb plays a dominant part. To be effective, fine sensory appreciation and tactile discrimination are required. The pattern of sensation present in the injured hand will determine the type of precision grip used. The right and left hands should be regarded as complementary to each other and ideally of equal importance, although in most persons one of them will be the dominant member.

The function of the normal hand is so complex that further, analysis, becomes artificial and therefore, of little value. In considering the mutilated hand, however, a classification of the basic requirements is helpful in planning treatment to achieve one or more particular aims. A hand devoid of movements and sensation is of no practical value. The presence of digits, conferring movements may allow the hand to work as a hook, to grasp or to punch. A hook is independent of the thumb but requires one or more fingers to be controlled in flexion even though the range of movement may not be great. For grasp to be effective at least 2, and preferably 3, fingers are necessary together with power of active flexion. Efficiency is greatly increased if the thumb is included. Pinch is characteristic feature of the thumb and is performed by its opposition to tip of the fingers or to any portion of the fingers or to any portion of the palmer surface of the hand which it is able to contact. In the normal hand, the index pulp is most frequantly used for this purpose but its function can effectively be taken over by the middle finger. By virtue of the arrangements of tendons already described, the index and little fingers have greater freedom of independent movement than the middle and ring but the disability following their loss is less. Amputation of either of the central digits causes a gap in the hand which is awkward functionally and noticeable cosmetically, whereas the work of the ablated index or little finger is taken over by the neighbor and the hand still appears (normal) neutral.

Position of Function

If the human hand is placed at rest, it takes up a certain position, this position of rest is also for most purposes the optimal position of function. The forearm is midway between full pronation and supination and the wrist is in about 15° of extension and 10° of ulnar deviation. All the Joints of the fingers are in an attitude of flexion which increases in amount from the index, which is a little less than half way between flexion and extension, to the little which is in rather more than this intermediate position. The thumb is partly abducted and opposed and also slightly flexed at each joint. This physiological posture is maintained by the normal muscles imbalance in the hand which depends on the interaction between three groups; the long flexors, the long extensors and the intrinsic muscles. Power is provided by the extrinsic muscles in the forearm and accuracy and steadiness by the small muscles in the hand. Injury to any one of these groups will upset the balance and may produce deformity.

The functional position determines also the functional range of movement. An example will make this clear.

30° of flexion at an interphalangeal joint is of much greater value if it is in the middle range of motion, than at either extreme. This applies more force to metacarpophalangeal (MP) joints, which cripple the hand if they stiffen in a position of hyperextension. It is obvious that these functional positions must be strictly observed during splintage some limitation of motion at one or more joints is anticipated. It is less obvious that they are important if full recovery is the aim. Rehabilitation is easier to achieve and active exercises are more natural in their performances; if each joint is in a resting position. Rigid immobilization and lively splintage should both be designed to serve this end.

Restoration of Hand Functions

For acute injuries of hand, restoration of function begins as soon as the patient comes under treatment, a surgical environment of efficiency and understandably is psychologically of great importance. Full cooperation on the part of the patient is the most important factor in the after rehabilitation.

Plaster Splintage

Plaster of paris (POP) plaster provides rigid immobilization during healing for the duration of some infective process in bone or soft tissue. Particular attention must be focused to ascertain that the fingers are adequately flexed at the MP joints, a point which is easily overlooked when plaster is applied over a layer of soft dressings.

Plaster correction is needed in the gradual restoration of the functional position when requirements of tendons or nerve suture have involved immobilizing the wrist fully flexed. It has also a special place in stretching adduction contractures of the thumb.

Lively Splintage

Its equivalent, is "Physiological Rest." As we understand it today, physiological rest is a controlled process which provides support to a part of the body while at the same time promoting restoration of function. It provides lively splintage and has following functions:

a. Support
b. Immobilization and limitation for movement
c. Correction of deformity
d. Mobilization of stiff joints
e. Substitution of defective muscular action.

These are based upon the principle of cock-up splints.

Occupational Therapy

The objective may be:

i. To assist physical rehabilitation by maintaining the normal patterns of functions and by active use to increase power and mobility.
ii. To re-educate the reconstructed hand and to adapt the mutilated hand to different patterns of movements.

First objective is best achieved by "Industrial" methods where by patient's work on simple machines adapted if necessary to suit particular purposes. It is desirable that such work should be productive.

The second aim is met by the traditional crafts associated with ocupational therapy. Such work must be creative and should involve hoth bands in simultaneous use.

Psychological Effects

There is frequently severe personality upset and dissociation with the injured hand particularly when this is the dominant one. The patient fatigues quickly and this is probably more psychological than physical. A rapid change of work will be needed, plus constant supervision and encouragement to make sure the hand is used, initially in any way that is possible. This is the most important factor in treatment. If he is allowed to delay his rehabilitation, he may never regain minimal functional ability and this should be made clear to him. The therapist may need to help the patient to overcome his fear of machines, electricity or what ever it was that caused his accident. This may prove impossible and resettlement in alternative work will be then necessary.

Activities of Daily Living

Problems of self-care are given priority. Some will be temporary but patient should be encouraged to wash, dress and use his knife, fork or spoon on his own. Grip may be inadequate to control tooth brush, razor, hair brush or pen. Handles may need to be adapted, with care to make them as unobstructive as possible, but as function improves normal grip will be expected to take over. Buttons usually done up with the injured hand, may be done by the other one, but an attempt should be made with the injured hand.

Edema

If possible, this should not be allowed to develop. When it is present or likely to occur, the hand should intermittently work in elevation. Active movements stimulate circulation and is beneficial for static muscles, work impedes it and is contraindicated. Gentle grip and release action on an overhead lever for drilling fulfills both the need for elevation and for movement.

Conditions of the Skin

The condition of the skin and any sensory loss should be checked before rehabilitation is begun. Wounds on the dorsum may open by movement and on the palmer surface may be traumatized by contact with tools or materials. Because early mobility is of prime importance, a delay in healing is justifiable, but if a small wound is opening into a larger one, medical advice must be sought. A crepe bandage will protect the palm but tubigauz, if necessary, covered with a Durex finger stall, will protect a finger scear tissue intricacies with elasticity of the skin and may tether it to underlying structures, for example scarring on the dorsum can prevent joint flexion. Rehabilitation must include skin toughening, especially when the patient is a manual worker.

Position of Wrist Joint

It is impossible to grip with the wrist in flexion and therefore, the optimum position is slight extension. If necessary, some form of cock-up splint should be provided. For a normal pattern of picking-up and release the wrist is in slight flexion and this should be the secondary aim. Flexion is also needed in many personal activities, particularly in washing and dressing.

Developing Span and Strengthening the Long Extensors

A good span is important because it is difficult to pick-up an object if the hand cannot spread over or encircle it first. The initial aim is to increase the thumb lost that is the distance between the joint heads of thumb and index finger and if possible to bring the thumb into opposition, then to increase the web between the little and ring finger because abduction of the little finger will increase the total span.

Increasing Metacarpophalangeal (MP) Joint

Flexion

This is necessary for all grips except hook grip. Precision punch grip, tip of thumb to tip of index finger, is impossible unless the index finger is mobile at the joint. When this joint is still, the thumb will pinch in adduction instead of opposition and this will not serve the same purpose. Rehabilitation activities include any pulling action with palmer grip, such as cross-cut sawing, a bench drill, or any squeezing action as in blow football. The palm must remain in contact in pulling it is easy to allow the hand to slip off the handle. Metacarpophalangeal joint flexion is also essential when exerting pressure between an opposed straight thumb and fingers with minimal interphalangeal joint flexion, as in picking-up draughts or 2.5 inch wide components for assembly work, holding a point fresh or the mesh stick for netting, pulling-up clay to make a pot. By substituting a handle 1.5 inch long for the normal one on a plane, or attaching one vertically to a polishing block, the little and ring fingers are responsible for the grip. This is also ensured by fixing a disk guard 1.5 inch from the end of the lever of a bench drill. To isolate responsibility to the index and middle fingers, the guard can be similarly fixed to a lever specially made with a crook-end.

Increasing Proximal and Terminal Interphalangeal Joint Flexion

This movement occurs in all digits in conjunction with metacarpophalangeal Joints flexion in cylinder grip and in all but the index finger in small tool grip. There is a partial flexion of the joints of the index finger and thumb during precision grip/work. It occurs in isolation in span and is solely responsible for hook grip. This is concerned with carrying shopping bags, buckets or books rather than "doing" and the thumb is not involved. To mobilize, these joints it may be necessary to block or immobilize the wrist and joints during rehabilitation. The flexors will act on the most mobile joints and when the wrist and metacarpophalangeal joints are flexed it is impossible to flex fully the interphalangeal joints as the travel of the extensor tendon will have been used up. Rehabilitation activities include many of those used for metacarpophalangeal joint flexion with palmer grip but by positioning the tool in lhe hand to use hook grip instead. Other activities using this grip are holding a dowel and using it either to work and adding machine or with an attached rubber stamp, cutting by pulling the knife towards the body, using pliers with a quick release spring, using spannar, peeling potatoes, whittling wood with a pen-knife; and picking-up playing cards by booking the finger tips underneath one side while stabilising the opposite side with an opposing thumb.

Re-education of the Pinch Grip

This grip may be a light picking-up action, thumb tip to index tip, it may be a stronger picking-up action, a tripod or three jaw chuck movement with thumb, index and middle finger, or it may be the more powerful key pinch between the thumb and the lateral side of the index finger.

Rehabilitation will include activities involving putting things into small holes and taking them out, picking-up and holding small objects by hand or with tweezers, as in printing, screwing of nuts or bottle tops, using paper clips, folding and tear paper, sculptures, clay modelling,

Re-education of Power Grip

Grips vary according to the article to be held and the purpose to which this will be put. Re-education of the grip will not be achieved when body weight or shoulder and elbows work are providing the main power, as for example, using a rip saw with a sawing horse but in a pulling action. as in cross-cut sawing, the muscles concerned with grip must do the work. Active gripping will be provided by a racket release mechanism on a lever handle. The resistance can be regulated mechanically, because the effect is not continuous and is suitable for repetition over a period of time. Continuous grip and release is required with metal slips; these must be held (with) in the hand, not in a vice. Resistance is regulated by the density of the material being cut but greater stamina is required and within a given period the muscles will be doing more work. Metal bending provides good static gripping exercise but body weight tends to undo the grip. Wedging clay provides both gripping action in gathering up the clay and forceful release action in throwing it down.

Work for Full-finger Extension and a Flat-hand

A stiff flexed finger will be knocked constantly. To begin with, assistance will be needed as the compatively weak finger extensors will be unable to overcome the joint stiffness or contracture for example, sanding or polishing with the injured hand on a block with a convex surface and the uninjured hand pressing down on the contracted joints.

Sensory Re-education

Compensation for the sensory loss is possible if there is some remaining sensation. The patient must learn to use the eyes instead or to feel with a different part of the hand, for example, using the ring finger instead of the index in a median nerve lesion. The therapist will try to re-educate stereognosis by, for example, getting the patient to handle coins, small objects such as pins and paper clips, and different materials without looking at them. When there is sensory loss, activities of daily living and work activities may present problems which will need attention.

Relating Rehabilitation to Patients Work

Rehabilitation is aimed not only at achieving maximally functional hand in general term, but the one which enables the patient to return to his particular job, for example, a touch typist may be incapacitated because she has residual stiffness in one little finger.

Limited aims of Rebahilitation where there is Gross Destruction

When there is inability to gain opposition of the thumb because of lack of abduction, try to get pinch grip against the PI joints of the index finger by working for thumb extension and adduction. Try to use any sensory area to the best advantage.

Assessment for Reconstruction

Assess function in relation to activities of daily living (ADL), work and recreation. Find out what tasks cannot be done and why they cannot be done? Refer this information back to the patient's surgeon and with his help, think in terms of aids and prosthesis which could be of value.

Media of Treatment

Because the hand is an indifferentiated instrument which is used in many ways, unlike the foot, which is specialized and consequently easier to re-educate, rehabilitation must be planned to give a repaid change of occupation. This is very necessary to avoid fatigue. It is also important and/in teaching the patient to use the correct pattern of movement at all times, not just on one piece of apparatus during rehabilitation. The occupational therapist must have a battery of activities from which she can select a suitable program.

Generalized Activities

The department should provide bilateral activities, sedentary and otherwise, suitable for women and men, during which the limbs will be used in a variety of ways, for example, woodwork, gardening, cooking and modelling. These will be an invaluable form of rehabilitation in the following circumstances. When an indirect approach is needed to draw attention away from the injured part, when there is need to improve the circulation throughout the limb prior to a period of specific local rehabilitation involving only small muscles; when an antidote is needed to the physical and mental fatigue which can result from repetition of difficult localized movements; when opportunity is needed for the patient to take some responsibility for his rehabilitation and when the therapist is unable to give him individual, specific attention.

Activities with Special Emphasis

Increase of Range of Movement (ROM)

By exerting maximum muscle power over a limited joint range to perform a movement that can just be managed with difficulty; for example, using a softly padded handle to facilitate grip (but thin padding must be used as flexion improves, otherwise it will be impending improvement rather than assisting it).

Increase of Muscle-strength

This will be mainly concerned with flexion; extensors rarely need strengthening. Stool seating, using a shuttle or a needle, needs a powerful grip.

Increase of Stamina

Is less of a problem than in the lower limb. The shoulder will tire more quickly than the hand. Blow football is excellent for improving stamina.

Increase of Speed

Is mainly necessary for those returning to repetitive production line work.

Increase of Dexterity

And the ability to perform fine finger movments which inevitably concern the thumb mainly involves tip to tip work and does not necessarily require full-range of movement, i.e. in rhematoid arthritis.

Work for the Nondominant Hand

It is unrealistic to try to exercise an injured nondominant arm or hand without considering whether the tool concerned is suitable.

Competitive Activities

Blow football, fair ground games, party games and cards are excellent for hand injuries because they can be adapted to provide movements that are difficult to isolate, such as pronation and supination or opening out the hand and throwing.

Thus, we find that hand gets the best all round care, as far as its full return to function is concerned, in the hands of occupational therapists. It is very truly said that function begets function in occupational therapy.

APPENDIX 12: OCCUPATIONAL THERAPY STUDENT'S CLINICAL PERFORMANCE FEEDBACK

For success of any professional pursuits is the skill required in performance of the concerned person. So is applicable to the professional of occupational therapy. Any occupational therapist who performs his/her functions in practice of this science become the determinant of the utility of the professionals to the society who suffer some or other kind of the disability.

The qualified occupational therapist who when gets into any job/ employment in any organization/institution or hospital or center, often likes to do away with documentation of services being offered by him/her in that organization. It has been world over felt in this area of therapy management and care that recording, evaluation, assessment of the cases under the occupational therapists (OTs) care generally are not properly recorded and documentation of such records is shirked by practicing occupational therapists (OTs). If documentation of records is shirked and services not kept properly, it will be very difficult for the treating occupational therapist to keep track of the progress/follow-up, etc. of his/her case.

But the question, arises what causes shirking of documentation in occupational therapists (OTs)? it is understood that due to growing needs of this professional service day by day growing disability incidence in the world, each therapist thus may be catering to patients in his/her department daily in between from 100 to 120 or more in some instances, where the organization is easily accessible to the disabled. This gives imperative answer to poor documentation of services in occupational therapists by occupational therspists that they hardly get time to do justice to documentation of treatment, progress and managements notes on case sheets or case files of these cases. So thus practising occupational therapists have evolved the method to write very very brief notes about cases and in some instances they only depend on their visual observations from time to time for the cases under their care.

When under such circumstances, the student trainees work under their senior teachers/supervisors, etc. at places of their clinical training becomes a model of learning for them. It is a point where the need arises that future generation of this profession does not pick-up these for their professional performance later in life.

Then how to achieve it? perhaps all the teachers and practising occupational therapists will agree here that less time consuming proformas, evaluation methodologies, etc. need to be evolved that documentation of services record of occupational therapy in respect of each case is properly kept for future reference, progress notes, treatment, etc. Hence need to computerized documentation is necessary for storing of the evaluation notes, treatment notes with diagnosis, progress notes, follow-up, etc. in any properly conducted occupational therapy department, it saves time but keeps proper records with minimum effort. While extensive use of computerized care of the cases is being taken in many advanced countries, perhaps it is now high time in this country also we think on those lines. Such an effort has been made at the occupational therapy school and center of my organization to make occupational therapy services in department more methodical, systematic and advanced in care and management to rate and assess functional performance efficiency in cases of disabled after every interval (when felt necessary) of administration of treatment in this department to see that human performance standards have been achieved after disability care in above department or not. This equipment is shortly under instalation in occupational therapy department of my institute.

There is also a proforma evolved by us which is filled by each student of occupational therapy who is placed for routine clinical training. The proforma has been evolved to be filled by the concerned occupational therapy. Trainee at the end of clinical posting (which is of one month duration) at occupational therapy department of the institute. The proforma is suggestive of the student trainees ability to learn different types of case evaluations, discussions on the treatment guide lines of the staff members under whom the each student is placed for that month.

The clinical proforma of students performance skills so evolved above, also is suggestive and reflective of the application of the knowledge in handling cases in occupational therapy department.

Also the type/number of evaluations each student of occupational therapy has learnt by heart.

Not only this, but also it was felt necessary by the institute that the teachers/supervisors of occupational therapy should also be exposed to various teaching methodologies so that quality teaching and training of these curricular courses is done. Many of occupational therapists may be already knowing or have participated in orientation course on teaching methodologies for occupational therapy teachers, which was organized by the institute nationaly for supervisors of occupational therapy to improve upon their instructional abilities for inducing good clinical and practice performance standards in occupational therapists.

The subject is vast which has more facets of its discussion. Due to time constraints it is not possible to discuss more. I thank the institute for the physically handicapped and the organizers of this conference without whom this publication would not have been possible.

APPENDIX 13: REACHING OUT TO THE RURAL DISABLED— AN OCCUPATIONAL THERAPIST'S VIEW POINT

Disability can fall on any one without considering caste, creed and religion. The population which is yet deprived of many technical advances is situated in rural parts of the country. The professionals generally like and wish to work in urban set-ups where there is already development of such services. The area which needs to be treaded thoroughly by professionals and technologists is the rehabilitation procedures and practices for the rural people.

The disabled, once disabled considers that his life has come to stand still. The person has number of questions in mind in context of his sickness and his prospects to overcome his disability. This often keeps the handicapped mentally and emotionally occupied. Thus affects his initiative drives to make an effort to cope with disability. This affects a great deal in functional rehabilitation of the disabled.

The total rehabilitation of any disabled person is dependent on the:

i. Economic condition of the concerned
ii. Social set-up from where he comes
iii. Type of disability he is suffering from
iv. Age of the disabled when he suffered from that particular illness
v. Educational background of the disabled.

It has been seen that. rural disabled are often lacking in the above prerequisites so need little more care by the occupational therapist in arranging and planning of their functional rehabilitation program to be as independent in activities of daily living as possible.

Occupational therapists has often to arrange such services in close liasion of the social worker or social welfare officer where ever she/he is working. The Institute for the physically handicapped is one of such examples.

This institute has various rehabilitation and treatment services for disabled of any age group, education facilities up to primary school level and bachelor degree courses for physical therapy and occupational therapy with a big workshop for orthotics and prosthetic for the handicapped. The institute is also an implementing agency for assistance scheme for the disabled of Ministry of Social Justice and Empowerment, Government of India. The scheme has only two categories to be entertained one who cannot pay and the other who can only pay 50 percent of the total cost of aid and appliances being distributed under scheme, Social workers help the poor cases to obtain affidavits and arrange money for aids, if necessary.

The above work is being looked after by an assessment team which evaluates the disabled cases from rural and urban parts of the country. Generally, the maximum beneficiaries are from rural India from various parts of the country. The social worker/social welfare officer after enquiry about the socioeconomic status contact various agencies/individuals/lion and rotary clubs, etc. to get financial aid to the disabled to get rehabilitation and treatment charges and related expenses for occupational therapy care are arranged by the social worker (SWO) of the institute as for other facilities of the institute also.

Many poor cases who undergo treatment in occupational therapy department of the institute or in other units are given the functional devices either free (if the case falls in that category) or social worker is informed in that case to raise or arrange funds for such poor cases to obtain any aid and appliance desired by him/her.

Some of the slides will show therapy being administered to such poor cases at the occupational therapy department of the institute or aids/appliances being fitted to the cases under financial assistance arranged by the social worker at the workshop of the institute.

While arranging camp along with team members conisting of occupational therapist, physiotherapist, vocational councilor, orthotician and prosthetician, speech therapist and social worker, the team assesses every poor/otherwise cases and also plans how to carry-out the program of therapy and fitments to rural disabled person.

These rural disabled are not only supplied with necessary aids and appliance but the occupational therapist with other team members ensures that the disabled becomes functionally independent as far as possible.

Follow-ups are also organized for disabled persons to see if the aids and appliances fitted on them are being really brought into use or he/she has only kept in their homes. During follow-up, if it is considered necessary, occupational therapist in consultation with the social worker helps scheduling of the treatment program and timings for treatment.

I feel that presence of the social worker in total rehabilitation program is very essential especially when working with socially deprived and economically backward cases in occupational therapy care. While concluding I may say that social worker is that part of the total chain of professionals in process of rehabilitation where treatment frame clutches to socioeconomic glue to make total program a grand success of rehabilitation even for the poorest of the poor.

APPENDIX 14: IMPROVING FUNCTIONAL ABILITY OF THE DISABLED THROUGH AIDS AND APPLIANCES

The functional freedom is very important to a disabled man. It enabled him to cope with day-to-day demands of living which otherwise would not allow him to do so. The achievement of functional freedom and ability is very big one for the rehabilitation team members and especially for an occupatonal therapist.

The lack of functional freedom can pose various kinds of the problem to the both disabled and the expert. If they are not over-come soon, might result into growing frustration in the mind of the concerned. Hence, the disabled requires training in enhancing his functional abilities either with the aids or appliances, if not achieved otherwise.

Although such a person may have a great deal of useful physical ability, the inability to perform one or more of the essential activities of daily living leaves him dependent on others. The dependence in self-care often prevents the disabled from returning to his home or holding a job. In many cases, no member of the family provides them with any assistance, they have to live as patients in the hospitals.

If handicapped wants to acquire a social status, he must be able to care for himself without any dependence on others.

In the course of each day each person must perform or be assisted in performing such activities as:

i. Arising from bed
ii. Caring for hygiene
iii. Eating
iv. Dressing
v. Using the wheelchairs
vi. Ambulation
vii. Performing vide variety of the manual tasks.

Any person who cannot do all these activities shall be dependent on others for daily tasks. In order to accomplish above tasks, any disabled person will require little or massive use of the aids/devices appliances as the case may be depending on the degree of limitation.

The Devices: Are provided to aid the disabled to easily perform activities like eating, dressing, combing, bathing and toilet activities.

The handles, the length of the rod required and to facilitate other easy hand functions, the need of effective devices becomes inevitable where further progress is not possible. These devices when prescribed are evaluated on the basis of demographic factors so as to asses their effective use and application.

The indications for the devices are in cases of:

   i. Lilmited range of motion in upper extremity

  ii. Poor hand function

 iii. Poor muscle strength

 iv. Nerve damages, etc.

Their effective prescription helps to obtain the desired functional efficiency results measuring their success. The objective mainly being in these prescriptions to improve manual dexterity which is very important aspect of accomplishing daily tasks successfully and properly.

There are a number of activities which encounter daily life than manual dexterity. Since performance of these activities is necessary for normal person, hence must be obtained independently in the disabled person also. Any patient who has impaired manual dexterity may have to use special techniques, special equipment or special procedures to accomplish that particular function.

The development of speed as well as precision of performance may be important in order to make the patient independent and vocationally productive in many instances.

Aids: Various kind of aids are advised for the disabled persons suffering from different kind of disability and functional problems.

The various aids which are generally used by the handicapped are:

- Wheelchairs
- Tricycles
- Stick
- Canes
- Crutches, etc.

These few, thus enumerated are major functional utility aids considered for the handicapped for achieving and improving their functional ability in ambulation and traveling from one place to another. The aids:

Wheelchairs: Are generally to move the disabled within his own house or little away from his home, etc.

Tricycles: Are used for traversing comparatively longer distances say few miles or so—these can be motorized or manual. But their prescription is on condition that disabled must have sound upper limbs.

Stick: Sticks are used by old people also. But the individual disabled with poor fracture healing, etc. also use them. They are used as means of partial support to the disabled. Some in case of fractures where full weight-bearing is not allowed as for leg fractures or other leg ailments where weight-bearing is to be avoided, the sticks are advised and prescribed. They are made to the size of the individual. Generally available in wood or aluminum.

There are other types of sticks also, out of which tripod stick is very commonly seen in use. The single tip stick slips due to lack of control on part of the patient, he falls or stumbles so tripod is advised.

Canes: Are also used like sticks but for short-term use only by those who desire support only in walking.

It is also said that canes and sticks should be provided to those where it become inevitable otherwise their use should be shirked as dependence becomes a problem later where the patient never tries to walk without support due to fear of fall or lack of initative to walk. They can also be of wood or aluminum as the case may be.

Crutches: Are more commonly known as "baisakhi in our day-to-day language of common man. These pair of crutches prove very important to those who are not advised weight bearing-partial or full, in case of one leg amputations, i.e. unilateral or in cases of severe leg deformities in case of one leg of the disabled.

These can be of bamboo/Jalneem wood or aluminium with its axillary pad well padded to come under the axilla to avoid any nerve damages arising out of excessive pressures thus caused.

Before the patient uses any kinds of prosthesis, etc. they enable the handicapped to make him move about independently.

Appliances: These are those which are applied on the person of the disabled. They are also very essential to obtain certain degree of functional freedom in the disabled persons. Their prescription has to be accurate, exact and minimal to its extent so as to avoid any discomfort being produced to disabled or affected individual. The various appliances can be catogrized as:

i. *Calipers:* Are provided to support the paralyzed leg or to prevent deformities in muscular dystrophy or nerve palsy cases of legs or to avoid weight on the paralyzed part.

These can be unilateral or bilateral with or without pelvic belt, with or without spinal support if spinal muscles are also weak. Other details like hip, knee and ankle locks will be advised as per needs of the individual case. The metal frame work is padded with leather. The leather straps used enable the proper fit of the caliper to the limb.

The shoes prescription goes in accordance with the rest of the caliper prescription.

Patient when wearing calipers in one leg, may not require crutches but may require later if wearing calipers in both the legs.

ii. *Splints:* The use of splints is for both upper and lower extremities as the case may be. There are various types of splints which can be static or dynamic. The static splints immobilize the part completely without any movement in the splinted part.

Whereas dynamic splints allow function as well as proper corrective support too. Therefore, they play a very vital role in achieving reasonably improved functional abilities in the disabled persons, they can be of plywood, soft wood, aluminium depending upon type of support desired. Their proper use at a proper time is really very beneficial to the disabled allowing him full or partial functional freedom.

iii. *Prosthesis:* The prosthesis are provided as replacement to missing parts of a limb or limbs as a whole. They are commonly, known as artificial limbs. These are of different types. Their effective and accurate prescription can do wonders in the life of the handicapped person.

In upper extremity, they are:

a. Above elbow prosthesis
b. Below elbow prosthesis.

In lower extremity, they are shown as:

a. Above knee prosthesis
b. Below knee prosthesis.

There are other kinds of the prosthetic fittings which will be determined by the age, sex, type of amputations, levels of the amputations, etc.

The prosthesis are fitted to the individual after obtaining his willing concent so as to promote his functional ability and his freedom in day-to-day life which causes him embarasment in a gathering or otherwise.

The individual who is prescribed unilateral or bilateral below or above knee or below or above elbow prosthesis must know well its application handling and management along with its maintenance, so as to enable him handle all minor repairs at home because visit to fitting centers only when there is major fault with his prosthesis. The utility limb is important to the wearer so therefore, the limb must not be exposed to sun heat/water excessively and deliberately by the concerned because it reduces the life expectancy of the gadget.

The prosthesis whether upper extremity or lower extremity involves very simple maneuvering techniques which can be learn by the patient without much difficulty. The patient should be tought to master the use of the prosthesis during his visit to the center for fittings.

iv. *Spinal supports*: They are the braces supporting spinal structures in correct position which get deformed/weak/diseased due to any cause. These spinal supports are commonly known as back supports to facilitate proper sitting, standing and walking. These can be prescribed alone or in association with calipers too. They are:

• Rigid
• Semirigid supports.

The selection of or either of the too above shall be determined by the extent condition, i.e. severity, etc. so that it should serve the purpose for which prescribed.

The rigid supports are either of PVC or metal reinforced to facilitate greater functional mobility. These can be padded with sponge or felt, solf leather-linning, etc. with leather straps, shall do what is desired. They are corrective in addition to suportive also.

The semi rigid supports are those which are not very firm, i.e. Canvas supports which acquire shape according to the contors of the body of the wearer. Therefore, they are not very much corrective but only supportive.

The different kinds of the spinal supports will determine the variety of prescriptions and range of service they render to the experts of rehabilitation.

Concluding, this can be stated that these aids and appliances have certainly a definite role to play in improving the functional abilities of the disabled persons.

APPENDIX 15: STUDENTS CONTRIBUTION IN PREVENTING ROAD ACCIDENTS

Occupational therapy in school setting is a known model of practice of (OT) in the world. Authoress widened the jurisdiction of the concept by involving the secondary school level children of willingly wished to come forward in our effort jointly with road safety cell of Delhi traffic police. This was not at all a difficult task as both schools and Delhi Traffic Police department were very keen on the thought to prevent accidents by careful driving.

The procedure is that school is identified by Delhi traffic police. The school children with their teachers are addressed by Dy Commissioner of traffic police on importance of safe driving and prevention of accidents. After this I am asked to address on the various accidental types of injuries, the problems arising out post-accident injuries and management of temporary or permanent injuries to these persons. The total emphasis of the task above is to make these teenagers and youngsters aware of various hazards of the accidents which can affect individual mentally and physically also.

These talks are motivational in nature to curb speed and respect traffic laws and regulations so as to teach these school children to be sensible drivers on road when they grow up as citizens. After these talk sessions, there is free discussion session with DCP and the authoress where both children and their teachers can ask any questions on this subject. The school managements make it a regular activity of their school children to assist traffic police constables/staff on the traffic intersections near or functionally convenient to them where their children assist in controlling traffic with traffic constables and a whistle.

These children perform regular traffic duties as and when possible. Children educate road users on traffic and road safety rules when traffic haults at red lights. Delhi traffic police believes that involvement of children at young age will be useful to make them aware of the hazards of negligent and rash driving by them before and after they attain the age of 18 years.

The above scheme is named as "CATCH THEM YOUNG." In addition to above the mobile van for road safety education has been commissioned at a cost of ₹ 11,00,000/— which is filled with every detail possible for the projection of the road safety films, rules regulations and skills required to drive to safety on road to prevent injuries from road accidents. On red light signals, these children educate the scooter, car, truck, taxi and auto drivers, etc. Even the pedestrians are trained as to how to cross road, from where and how and when to cross roads.

The culture of stopping vehicles on stop line is also developed so that pedestrians can cross the road safely when red signal is there. This is done by school children under the duty staff of the traffic police where possible, authoress also joins them.

Even Delhi University NSS students volunteers are also providing road safety education to the road users and any vehicular drivers including pedestrians. As authoress is commissioned at A-point of ITO which is the busiest traffic crossing of Delhi where about 30 to 40 thousand or more vehicles pass everyday, have many times transported the accident victims to nearby emergency of Lok Nayak Hospital which is a state Government run big Genenral Hospital with associated GB Pant Hospital, New Delhi.

Sometimes road users volunteer to take accident victims to the hospital and also some volunteers use their mobile phones to inform the families of the victims of the accident. To provide on the spot guidance or vehicle assistance in case of any accident, Delhi police petrol vans also come forward for the victims.

Like this children are made aware of their involvement into the prevention of accidents and on the disabilities arising out of accidents. The children are also associated with various "Road safety week" celebrations every year in the month of January, when exhibitions are inaugurated at Pragati Maidan. Traffic pavilion with traffic training park is also thrown open to general public for getting educated on road safety and prevention of accidents leading to disabilities through audio-visual films which are in English and Hindi both so as to impart message of preventing accidents including avoiding drunken driving also.

Note: An effort is being made with Delhi traffic police to make possible to show a video film of the same.

In the end, I would like to say that occupational therapists have numerous ways to act professionally with better care given with a motivation and spirit to pay back the ex-checker to whom each one of us owes in the form of service to the community, society and the nation to which we all ought-to while submitting unabatedly and always. Do what ever you can, in your way, to contribute your effort to further the cause of occupational therapy—commitment to service-our professional pride.

APPENDIX 16: OCCUPATIONAL THERAPY IN 2000—A PERSPECTIVE

Occupational therapy has diversified itself in so many areas that it is very limited explanation to justify its gamut of catering to the various types of disabilities.

Though, this profession has considerably developed into the area of Physical disabilities more than in the areas of psychiatry and mental health including mental subnormality and drug abuse.

In present times, occupational therapy is not coming into full picture of its potential use in functional rehabilitation of different disabilities. There are far less occupational therapists who are working in the area of psychiatry and mental health including subnormality. Thus, the logical conclusion from the various previous conferences is that we hardly have contributions on role of occupational therapy in mental sub normality, psychiatry including drug abuse. However, drug abuse have found certain attention from government, institution, families and the addicts themselves. There are numerous institutions/organizations which either have no occupational therapy or post is lying vacant for want of an occupational therapy (OT). Almost similar picture we see in the area of Psychiatry also. There are hardly any occupational therapists (OTs) who are doing good work in this field with psychiatric cases. We need to motivate occupational therapists (OTs) so that more and more occupational therapists (OTs) join psychiatry area for occupational therapy practice and where there is no competition with any other co-professional. Same holds true in Mental subnormality too. But to surprise there is extra congestion in the area of physical disabilities. This needs to be taken care' of so that vacant posts in the areas of psychiatry, mental subnormality and drug addiction, etc. are filled.

There is a lot to be done in creation of posts of occupational therapists (OTs) in various institutions/organizations. This can be looked after with proper media publicity, through awareness camps, through work in near by colonies where incidence of disabilities is there.

All the practising occupational therapists give improper identity in some cases which affects popularity of this profession adversely. The use of proper occupational therapy skills in functional training aspects needs an effort before discharging any patients either from hospital/institution/center.

It has been observed that some of the occupational therapists (OTs) do not evaluate cases at regular intervals which leads to poor documentation of cases and their management as well as treatment details.

The energy conservation methods are highlighted in the proper discharge of the services towards the disabled persons but not in documentation.

As has been often observed that occupational therapists (OTs) who are working in General hospitals/institutions where out patient load is on an average from 80 to 120 cases per day, the therapists straight away start the modality treatment even without evaluation of the case. It appears incorrect because there are no two cases alike pathologically. It is, therfore, very essential to evaluate each case first and them start actual treatment of that case. There needs to be a moral responsibility where patients, views are also respected in such a manner that later is also a party to his/her management under the therapist who is managing the case.

It is considered necessary that each occupational therapist does not start treatment without evaluating a case.

Other areas to be of importance are forensic occupational therapy where it is important for legal aspects of practice of any profession so that legal implications of any professional actions need to be addressed fully before harming oneself innocently and be implicated. Most of the occupational therapists due to unawarness of legal implications of their practice harm themeselves.

Consumer Protection Act has come into force because of such lapses in the medical practices which has been made now compulsory in the jurisdiction of the practitioners of any professional service.

Industrial therapy is also an important vital area of the practice of this profession. At present, the big business houses are not mostly having establishments of this kind for the welfare of their employees and their family members. The health hazards due to accidents on job sites and use of chemicals in some industries. These types of situations make it imparative to have facilities for occupational therapy attached to industrial set-ups with or without a hospital set-up.

This area needs an extensive effort for creation of posts for occupational therapists which not only improves the occupational health of the concerned worker but also improves his efficiency a lot. I propose here that AIOTA should take an initiative to correspond/ meet with officials of Ministry of industries or labor if so desired.

Due to restricted employment policies in the western countries, we need to think to creat more avenues in various types of industrial set-ups where employment facilities could be created all over the country through central government machinery. This we need to consider for every training school of occupational therapy to train occupational therapists in as many numbers as possible by opening proper training establishments for occupational therapists (OTs).

Another area which needs a greater emphasis is the area of the functional training of the disabled cases which occupational therapists come across. There is lot of need of functional training occupational therapists because when any occupational therapy manages a case during treatment settings, generally it is seen that remedial occupational therapy is administered and after obtaining results, the case is dischrged. Where as no case should be discharged til he/she is able to perform functional activities independently.

Thus, there are many other areas which need to be explored for penetration of the professional skills of the field of occupational therapy. The millinium hopes are the thoughts of professional development and growth for the interest of each occupational therapist.

APPENDIX 17: SPORTS AND RECREATION FOR THE PHYSICALLY AND VISUALLY HANDICAPPED

Sports and recreation have a significant effect on mind and body of human beings. The values of the two are manifold which could be satisfaction of the personal needs, personality development/physical well-being, emotional well-being, social interaction, etc. All these clubbed together make mind and body rich within body resources of a person.

These two, i.e. sports and recreation have equal importance as above in the field of the rehabilitation of the physically handicapped and visually handicapped. The recreation/sports may need, certain adaptations in their application in visually and physically handicapped persons. These adaptations could be in the various areas on the play fields. Hence we may call it therapeutic recreation affecting mind body and performance of a person.

The challenge of the therapeutic recreation is also there. There are many individuals who due to variety of circumstances, are unable to fulfill their social responsibilities or benefit from the concomitant effects of recreation and its experiences. These individuals get a key through these means to self-discover themselves while unlocking their personality, or to self-respect or to the joy of sharing interests amongst themselves with experiences of others clubbed with their own.

Some population segment consists of those who are affected by some form of physically or mentally incapacitating disease or disability, old age, poverty, socially deviant behavior and institutionalization. These physically handicapped and visually handicapped persons society have their interest and needs also like normals—self expression, social involvement and creative experience.

We just cannot afford to deny these persons the opportunities to participate in the recreational life of the nation even though participation may be limited. The important experience of recreational avenues is opened where ever possible. We are perhaps doing a great deal towards mental and physical development of these categories.

Recreational experiences through sports and other means of recreation provide an excellent opportunity for the handicapped to associate informally with society as a whole. Those experiences can contribute to the rehabilitation of the handicapped persons and their inclusion in education, employment and other individual social functions.

Just as public hygiene is concerned with the health of the people who are well as much as with the illness of those who are sick, so recreation has implications for everyone. In its broadest sense, the aim of leisure and recreation service is to help all persons achieve fuller, happier and more harmonious and effective lives.

A constructive attitude to life is important to each person, the recreative experiences can contribute to such an attitude. The professionals should realize that they are in a position to help this segment of population/society to progress towards better physical, emotional, social, and intellectual adjustment through recreation. Thus we see that the recreation gives an opportunity for a growth of a person as a whole. Various sports are varieties of ways in which the recreation could be possible and assist in progress towards better physical emotional, social and intellectual adjustment through recreation.

As denial of recreation in many instances is a challenge of therapeutic recreation as a helping profession. The general segment of this prey is disabled person, social offenders, disadvantaged persons, etc.

Who most often need these services are in two categories of factors:

a. Health producing
b. Disease producing.

Health Producing

Health producing factors are good hereditary endowment, healthful safe environment, adequate service and education, resistance to communicable and noncommunicable diseases, optimum dynamic soundness and functional vigor, optimum dynamic motor fitness and suitable exercise throughout life, refreshing rest, relaxation and sleep, resistance to stress, fatigue, frustration and boredom, healing, repair and recovery from injury or illness, resistance to premature aging and death, healthy mature personality with healthful living. A well to live, healthful beliefs and attitudes and practices, freedom for personal-social fulfillment through significant commitments to ultimate concerns, useful, satisfying creative work achievements, love and affectionate sharing and belonging, heterosexual adjustment, enjoyment of constructive recreation and use of leisure, enjoyable esthetic experiences including those with nature, opportunities for risk, challenges, adventure and new experiences, spiritual faith, ideals, values and a search for meaning.

Disease Producing

The disease producing factors are just opposite to listed above. The rehabilitation punishment is to totally curb such facilities for this category of our brothering of society. The various ways of recreation and recreation through sports as applied will depend upon the disease of which one is suffering and type of the disorder one is suffering from.

Effective human efficiency is dependent upon the smooth function and integration of bodily parts and various systems including musculoskeletal, cardiovascular, respiratory, digestive, genitourinary, endocrine, nervous and reproductive systems. One cannot alter one organ without bringing changes in others.

Implementation of sports and recreation for physically and visually handicapped is and should be taken care of at the various agencies and institutional levels, where government could be approached for certain limited funds to club with organizational resources.

Such activities should be taken care of most of the time by professional agencies and nongovernment organizations. The professionals like occupational therapists and physical therapist can also contribute a lot towards this as they have knowledge of various mind and body disorders, and these two modalities of sports and recreation can be used therapeutically as discussed.

APPENDIX 18: PROSPECTUS OF DEVELOPMENTS OF OCCUPATIONAL THERAPY IN INDIA AND ABROAD

The profession of occupational therapy is being felt as a solution to the problem of the disabled of any kind. This has become possible due to its versatility of applications in any condition, disorder, age, sex and status of the case. The advances in technology have also catered to occupational therapy skills through the extensive use of computers in its software developments and in documentation of records of the patients and their case sheets and reviews from time to time.

Whenever any developments account is taken, we need to see its growth in the field of the professional education.

   i. Facilities provided for training for the professionals in that field.

  ii. The government and state government and statute bodies breathing with the attitudes of the policy makers and planners of any country.

     a. The root level options to work in the area of disability.

     b. The enthusiasm, keeness, willingness, initiative of the professional and the professionals of that field.

With a scanning view of the account of some aspects of the list above, we see that each one of the above is important in its own right.

Computers have invaded almost every sphere of human life in its welfare, efficiency and stream lining of services even in occupational therapy.

The foreign developments can account for in various areas of practice and training.

In various areas in which occupational therapy is employed in various countries are manifold as in community, forensic model, indoors as for four walls of an institution/center/organization.

The service catering is little deficient on account of availability of the manpower at disposal in the country. While caring for the welfare of the disabled category of the patients, therapists have opted to look to their own welfare too. I do not mean here that therapists should not look after themselves but it is happening so fast in my country that developments in India are being affected a great deal.

For the last many years, undergraduate courses were being conducted in many parts of the world, later on master level education started developing in many countries. In India, master education in occupational therapy is of very recent times. The affluent countries have PhD facilities because their senior professionals are available in their own countries and number of schools are present so far thesis guide problems does not arise. Whereas in my country PhD degrees will suffer in future for want of guides for postgraduates in occupational therapy in India.

In our country distant education facilities are hardly available. continuing education programs are also scarcely available. This is also the area where we need to think for the occupational therapists working in India. Perhaps it could be actively considered by AIOTA in coming years.

The profiles of current students and recent graduates to inspire to also participate in further study and research. The freeships/scholarships should be amply available to promote educational standards further in India. Sometimes, students find hardships to continue their studies at graduate or postgraduate levels.

The education is to enable you to gain the most from studies. There are a range of services and facilities which become prerequisite to acquire certain standards of education.

It is a high time, when we should promote and under take research in the areas of education and occupation. The word occupation is well inherent in OT. Occupation, i.e. a goal directed use of energy, time, interest and attention. The role of schools of occupational therapy in India is for identifying innovative projects, attracting funding and deliver valuable research products.

Public health and rehabilitation are very closely linked subjects which form an integral part of the total health care management system including women's health. Occupational (Vocational) health and old age persons health.

My rationale of this submission is:

1. New scientific developments in OT theory and practice must continue.
2. Need for research to assess and document effectiveness of OT should be continued.

3. Growing interest in assuring that OT meets the needs of a multicultural global community all over.
4. Changing practice environment has created new clinical, ethical and administrative challenges for professionals of OT.
5. Need for doctorally prepared OT faculty may be conceived for future in this country.
6. Need for clinical specialists with more advanced training in OT should be felt in India.

Like this, we see that there is no end of discussions on developments as discussed here in India and aboard but I limit it to this little submission due to time constraints.

APPENDIX 19: OCCUPATIONAL THERAPY AND CARDIAC RHYTHM

The heart can support activities which require different amounts of muscular effort in every human being. Oxygen is the main requirement for normal heart functions like any other muscle of the body. The blood carries O_2 to various tissues to keep them alive and active to perform functions.

An increase in work load will increase O_2 demand in body reflected by increased respiration. Less O_2 than the required amount in one given time increase O_2 debt in body reflected by breathlessness in any normal person.

The diseases like angina pectoris, myocardial infraction, angina anomalies if any, hypertension, A-V Block, ventricular tachycardia, uncontrolled atrial fibrillation, frequent premature ventricular contractions at rest which increase with exercise, cardiac enlargement, etc. are most commonly come across by any person working in the area of cardiac rehabilitation.

For effective management of these cases in occupational therapy these patients can be classified according to the amount of work and kinds of activities they can perform safely. The O_2 requirements are measured while performing ADL, recreational and vocational tasks.

Energy cost of activities can be valuable in determining the intensity of effort required by activities.

The cardiac cases can be classified on the basis of their functional abilities so its called *functional classification.*

The therapeutic classification will determine the classifying patients on the basis of their physical effort requirement and abilities.

For planning effective occupational therapy program for these cases, the points which influence the planning are:

  i. Type of muscular contraction
 ii. Posture in any activity
iii. Work rate
 iv. Anxiety if any in the concerned
  v. Stress requirement on body.

In addition to above, it is also observed that occupational therapist has to help the patient along with physician, nurse for better and effective OT care. She OT has to effectively explain the disability to the patient and to his family members for better understanding of patients own problems and the type of help and understanding required from the members of family. The program has to be made effective by careful explanations to the patient to change his elements of lifestyle, i.e. diet, smoking, reactions to stress and various habitual methods of relating to others. The psychiatric training of occupational therapy makes is/her suitable person to join team with psychologist or psychiatrist in enabling patient to relearn habits of dealing with stress and interacting with others.

Mainly OT program starts with light activities including self-care for the purposes of improving and increasing cardiac capacity there by decreasing anxiety and hence stress. The grading of the activities has to be in duration and also in the rate of the repetitions. These are interrelated so should be carefully handled. The intensity is most critical because it is the intensity that taxes the heart.

The training effect is seen for all activities within the classifications and may change the class in which he was at the start of the activity program.

Each activity session can start with warm-up period and end with a cooling off period. As for example, walking fast walking followed by jogging and end with fast walking and walking.

Stress testing (exercise testing) can be done by ascending and descending standard size and number of steps. This should be generally carried out in presence of cardiac physician to manage cardiac distress if any.

As tables are available to determine average maximum heart rate by age and sexes, the activity if need be can be controlled with such informations without any difficulty to the patient.

The patient is subjected to an activity in a standardized manner, beginning at a low intensity and progressing until fast heart rate is reached or any indications are there of over exertion.

Eightly five percent of the maximum heart rate for a given individual is called the heart rate.

The occupational therapists emphasis is on the planning which is graded progressively resistive depending upon his state of heart condition. Generally, an occupational therapy faces a face which shows an expression of concern if he would be benefited with that sort of activities planning in his case. Which needs an explanation from the treating occupational therapy so that the patient himself joins the therapist in his own objective achievements. This effort shown on the part of the patients goes a long way in future footing and base of occupational therapy program towards functional rehabilitation of these cases.

Suddenly light work activities in occupational therapy on bed and later on as the cases show improvement in functional capacity and abilities go to the extent of moderately assistive program outside bed in the department of the center or hospital.

It is suggested that activities like paper crafts, cane crafts, balsa crafts, cord crafts may be advised under supervision of the therapist who is closely monitoring the heart and other signs like sweating and dyspnea while patients are being engaged on any of the above activities.

The occupations like involving minimal physical effort should be prescribed by occupational therapy like lifting office files, handling supervisory jobs where much strain and effort is not required on the patients side. It must be remembered that a reasonably controlled craft activities program with necessary gradation in performance of drills, dramas, singing—group/chorus, etc. should be controlled and regulated under strict supervision.

It may be remembered always that each cardiac case needs a tailor made program in occupational therapy with result oriented targets. I would recommend that the cardiac cases if can be cured as quiet and tension free individuals, there is no more need of any planning but a sound heart on systematic rhythm of life for later years to come.

APPENDIX 20: OCCUPATIONAL THERAPY AND ADVANCE IN ENGINEERING

Engineering today is an integral part of life as it involves its advances in different trends of appliances/aids/machines, etc. which help a common man in day-to-day life.

The advances in the life of an individual can be fruitful both socially and mentally. Technological advances have become even integral part of medicine for generations. The engineers and physical scientists have made contributions to biological and medical knowledge since antiquity and physician and biologist have contributed to the advancement of the physical sciences.

As the health care delivery system has considerably evolved, engineers have continued to play a role and technology has been a major part of this evaluation. Although, the marriage of technology and health care has been strong at times, there have been significant advances and changes in the health care system brought about by technology.

Despite success in the past, many problems plague many modern health care systems. Some of these problems have roots in technological changes and other depend on technology for solution.

The historical overview shows that during the ninteenth century there were different systems and organizations. Showing different styles of practices. The present day practice shows that basic clinical investigations are dependent on role of instruments in diagnosis. When such advances showed its appearance in medical practice the appearance of such advances were also seen in other methods of therapies like oral therapy as well.

The advances in the manufacture of the goniometers resulted in an aid to measure joint range irrespective of they are small or big. This device to measure the joint movement is of tremendous use in planning the basic occupational therapy activities to facilitate early return to function and hence back to work.

The catheterization in heart diseases has helped improve heart efficiency in day-to-day function hence helping the disabled suffering from heart disease function more efficiently than without a device. This in the long run helps the disabled and the therapist to assess his functional capacity in occupational therapy modalities. This helps control and advice dosage of this therapy for the concerned patient to make him useful member again of society as before his illness.

Mechanical safety: It is one of the foremost components in delivery of the treatment in occupational therapy to the disabled. This can be looked after under following heads:

General design consideration of the equipment and machinery for that matter. The reason of this consideration is patient care and not instrument care, say for electrical equipment being used by the patient in occupational therapy department, if necessary safety is not provided in design consideration, may lead the patient and operator to injury during treatment process which further delays the rehabilitation of the cases.

The equipment abuse: One answer to it is problem of inadequate staff education to handle such equipments which instead of improving treatment program, may cause distortion in the treatment approaches.

Hence to handle such advanced technologies and engineering the necessary short-term courses for both therapists and the operator if possible should be conducted, so as to economize on effect in rehabilitation process and repairs of equipment/machinery frequently, due to management and handling abuse.

It is the time when we should think of evolving the mechanics of the different types of machines in occupational therapy department, which should be "Fail Safe Design" sort of thing which neither injures the patient nor line operator or therapist but provides a safety guard to injury during treatment sessions.

Tissues trauma: Tissues break own in the form of abrasion of the skin surface or pressure sores can occur as a result of pressure, sheer strains or torsion continuously on intermittently provided in for long sitting activities or short sitting activities requiring the use of fretsaw/treadle saw or bicycle fret saw machine. These might pose problems of gravity on if these tissues trauma get unchecked in the department settings or in hospital settings.

We may consider protection from tissue trauma in the form of breaking up of an activity process or time so as to minimize hazards later.

Patient Mobility Devices and Barriers

It is proposed that need to plan the training programs of short duration for the uses (patient) and the attendant be organized so as to facilitate hazard free mobility through:

a. Electrical wheelchairs.
b. Mannual wheelchairs.
c. Other mobility aids like canes, sticks, crutches and four legged walkers.
d. Mannual driving aids being used by the disabled also posed a challenge to the occupational therapists as the occupational therapists are the persons responsible to teach the functional freedom in mobility and use of such devices which provide early independent mobility.

General Building Safety

In the present times of advances in civil engineering has faced a considerable challenge in providing a barrier free building to the disabled. To achieve total functional freedom in such kind of a building calls for an occupational therapist to train a person in that advanced constructed building in full functional activities to the disabled so that he does not require any assistance from any person or attendant.

Like this there are various other aspects where the advances of the engineering are a boon, and also pose threat simultaneously.

Since it is an on going process we the personnel's responsible have to keep pace with advance of engineering technology and go on finding solutions to problems thereafter such advances.

APPENDIX 21: NEED FOR LEGISLATION FOR ACCESS: PARTICIPATION OF GOVERNMENT

The disabled has been taken care of at every front of the phase of their lives by various government and semi government along with voluntary organizations in their rehabilitation into the main stream of their lives in the recent times.

There has been considerable contribution of the Central and State Government in the various existing rules/regulations pertaining to the lives of the disabled of varied kinds.

There is reservation of jobs, allotment of houses, shops, booths, kiosks, etc. to the handicapped persons giving status to them like any one of us. This is the policy of equality of the disabled with any other normal citizen of the country.

There is yet an area where we need to dwell and ponder the legislation for access. There are some construction, design and building laws for different kinds of the buildings to be constructed for different purposes in the country, there should be specified laws which should be incorporated in the existing laws to promote easy access to all the types of the buildings being constructed in the nation where there is disabled population also a user of the same.

It will not be out of place to state here that I know of a building which houses activities for the disabled, the beneficiaries are implied disabled and not able to move around the building freely because in one block ramp has been provided up to first floor only. There is no ramp in the block where the disabled have to go for advice and making changes of the treatment.

It is emphasized through this example that we must provide ramps invariably in all the building reaching to the top floors with staircase also running parallel to the ramps. It is stated further that if need considered, we may amend building construction and design laws for such provisions.

The toilet designs should be such that it must have the railing (firm fittings) on the walls at standard heights for holding in case of the ataxies, cerebral palsied, quadriplegics and paraplegics who will come with wheelchairs. The minimum standard size of the corridors, doors, toilets seats, toilet doors and wash basin areas inside toilets should be friendly wheel chair friendly. The corridors should invariably have railing fixed in two different heights firmly so that the disabled can move about unassisted where ever possible in the building where they have to be for the service, work and employment.

It is the need of the hour to incorporate a clause that it is essential to have each and every building invariably being constructed with easy and free access for the disabled. I will not agree to the argument that it is not possible because those who are normal do not know what is in store for them in future. Therefore, my suggestion should we the ponderers have to have the thought estimates for future needs as well.

No shopping complex should be designed, constructed and built without easy access for the handicapped. When we strive to give them functional freedom—It becomes inevitable that each building, shopping complex, restaurant, club, sports stadiums indoor or open air, cinema halls, race courses, houses, hospital, government/semi government offices, factories, mills, etc. should have easy access to these places for the disabled persons.

There is only one way to achieve that legislation to this effect. No building should be given fitness certificate at any cost if it does not provided easy access for the disabled persons as I would like to appeal to the authorities who issue fitness certificate to each constructed building. It is only this much that needs to be done.

Due to time constraints, I have made some effort to bring some of the thoughts to this platform for consideration at length while delebrations/recommendations will be sent to government and other related departments.

APPENDIX 22: OCCUPATIONAL THERAPY AS A TREATMENT MEDIUM

We all know that there is lot of contribution of occupational therapy to the service of suffering mankind for quite some years in the past and also trying to contribute at present with steady stride to innovations in future to improve quality service to the disabled.

Social critics are emphasizing the dramatic changes that we are beginning to experience in our society. All technical, economic, scientific with social forces are combining to reshape and restructure our worlds.

Many traditional institutions will change in response to those transformations in society. The same provokes the transforming role of occupational therapy in that perspective in total health care delivery system to masses of our country.

The need of the hour is to take therapy service to door step as far as possible so as to make disabled have benefit of the science of activity and craft to enable them regain their functional skills towards normalcy.

The therapy by occupation as we know is an important mode of application of the treatment in modern times of today to mentally and physically sick individuals.

The role of occupational therapy is largely contributing to functional freedom to the disabled. As we see in the past and even in recent past, it is observed that this mode of therapy was more or less was confined to four walls of the departments.

Keeping in view, the revolution in the field of technology and medical world it has given impetus to carrying of rehabilitation services to the door steps of the disabled who actually need these services. This is only possible when we review the applicability of this science in prespective of technological advances which may also be understood in terms of carrying the occupational therapy services outside institutions. This may be only possible when occupational therapy is rural based and in rural set-ups with all the materials available in that particular rural population.

For encouraging such type of establishament, various preliminary excercises are required such as:

i. Disability survey
ii. Lifestyle of the inhabitants of that particular rural population
iii. Incidence, type, classified disability range
iv. Educational background on an average
v. Socioeconomic status on an average there and so on.

While concentrating on the functional restoration part of this particular therapy skill, it becomes obvious that actively involved limbs in the performance of any kind of activity shall determine the utility of this therapy to restore the capacing of the concerned in the lost skills.

The involvement of the therapist should determine the content of the applied therapy to bear the desired results to fuller functional rehabilitation. I may add here that in the not too distant future individuals will be able to benefit both physically and psychosocially from startling technological advances.

The invention of solar cookers, biogas plants, etc. are perhaps proof of rural technological advances towards that style of life. I may say that perhaps a reasonably good percent of the burn cases may not now occur with solar cookers in use which has gone far to save the housewife from such kitchen accidents.

We may also note that high technological advances will offer adaptive lifestyles to those with developmental disabilities.

Many of the services will be derived from the health services already being provided in the country.

It is said that situation is different when the human system is involved primarily because humans grow and change rather than simply maintain function, people develop highly refined and specialized skills as they interact with their environments.

The individuals are "open systems" in that they are capable of acquiring and using information from their environment and most importantly, and they control their behavior internally.

It is a characteristic of a system that there is interaction among its various parts, so that changes in one part are likely to have considerable consequences in several other parts. A system, furthermore, tends to maintain itself as intact as possible and thus displays more or less extensive rebalancing process when injured or deformed.

Everyday advances in the field of science are exposing human body to bear brunt of occupational hazards thus leading to disablement of different varieties.

It becomes all the more necessary that a constant regular review of the skills of occupational therapy in context of the developments in all spheres is made to meet the required demands of time from time to time.

APPENDIX 23: OCCUPATIONAL THERAPY: MAKING NEEDED CHANGES

The transformation in thinking and problem-solving is a long standing and familiar orientation to occupational therapists. As early as 1910, occupational therapy embraced the recognition that an individual's health was bound up in the intricacies of daily experience in a complex and social world. This science got organized around the concept of occupation and profession has from its beginning, using notions of self-satisfaction in daily living, balance in work, play, sleep and rest mastery and competence, learning through activity and practice for real life situations—as the underpinnings of treatment.

Disease and disability have always been viewed as disruptions in a person's life and the goal of intervention has always been to re-establish habits and skills that would insure a person's return to a satisfying life. This has always been the concern of occupational therapists.

In 1980s and beyond, survival of occupational therapy is not dependent, on our ability to change our way of thinking from mechanistic a systems view. We have always treated the person as a whole. The treatment procedures and plans are based on factors like interest, values, goals of the plans of the treatment.

In a sense, more than even, occupational therapy is an idea whose time has come. The long standing professional expertise that we all possess in occupation and associated areas that include recognition of the importance of survival skills, the relationship between curiosity and activity are the basis for intervention strategies that insure an individuals adaptations to the environment.

Our survival as a profession depends more on our ability to act quickly and effectively in response to the changing needs and environments in health care.

The service occupational therapists provide is vital today and will be in even greater demand in the future. The greatest challenge to occupational therapy lies in our ability to communicate what we do and how our service will benefit people, their family and society.

APPENDIX 24: FUTURISTIC DEVELOPMENT OF OCCUPATIONAL THERAPY—INDIA

I feel that there is no profession in this universe which does not ever have future development plans. It is as inevitable as anything else that the future development has to begin one day. Then why wait further, lets thing to start just now—this very minute.

We all know that occupational therapy is the science of healing through occupation which can be very creative, original, novel and practical way to achieve ones results while administering this therapy. Not only this, it is also said that to tread on any beaten path also is not the principle of this versatile branch of physical medicine in rehabilitating the disabled of various kinds and types in our society.

The science of practice of occupational therapy, has thus made the occupational therapy not less than a computer to produce know how to achieve objectives of treatment in any individual case of the disabled being looked after by any qualified occupational therapy in a hospital/department/center/home where ever one is employed to look after the functional rehabilitation and training needs of that particular organization.

I, as a practitioner of occupational therapy, as teacher of occupational therapy feel that being in the field of occupational therapy for the last two decades that we the occupational therapists have yet to contribute more towards the community at large.

The contributions which we can make can be like:

To provide extension facilities in training and treatment of the handicapped from the place where one is employed: At present what I see the catering is only in the four walls of the department or more to the wards in case where the occupational therapy is in hospital set-ups.

While extending services to catering of occupational therapy from department it can be the other voluntary/private agencies by us to help them set-up occupational therapy departments inside their set-ups. We can depute one occupational therapy daily to treat their patients whosoever need the services of occupational therapy towards fuller functional rehabilitation. Thus we are bridging the gap of practicing occupational therapy and his parent organization to have a proper communication towards better health care and relationship. Also those disabled who needed services but were not getting due to lack of facility of occupational therapy get their due share of attention. Thus, we widen the scope of the services in occupational therapy for better utility are increasing the number of beneficiaries in the same expenditure.

Postal consultancy/advice facilities: I have seen in two decades of my being in field that the practicing/teaching/training personnel's also do this invariably. We will not only reach to those who come to our door step of occupational therapy department avail of our attention, care and facilities but there are many who on any account/reason are neither able to bring the patient to our department nor can they afford to have a private occupational therapy to visit them at home to treat them and charge for such a visit. What is needed is that we may form a common point wherever occupational therapy departments are existing in the hospital/centers/institutions that such postal advice services are advocated and more publicized in case of those who just cannot come to your department or are not financially sound to have you as a private occupational therapy for visits at their respective homes.

Easy to do home management kits: Such kits should be deviced by occupational therapists for those disabled persons who are going to live with their disabilities for life times. These disabled persons who need to go back to their original/previous jobs (must be sent at all costs) if occupational therapy is convinced of the case that he/she is now functionally fit to go to the same job. It will be perhaps the best.

In cases, where the disabled persons are not able to go to any kind of a job because they are so crippled then such kits should help them to look after their own needs at home for the purpose of feedback and follow-up the concerned occupational therapy may remain in touch of such cases monthly/fortnightly as the case may be till she is convinced that she can now detach herself from the concerned care.

Community education by Occupational Therapists: I have to my information that there is hardly any emphasis by the practitioner of occupational therapy that take-up the role of education of community. The community education will be useful on the following aspects, namely.

Disability awareness and its hazards: This can be by way of arranging camps, exhibitions, film shows and distribution of pamphlets which give the community the information why disability should not occur, how should it be managed and taken care of and how and where.

I may not hesitate to add here that this proves useful to a great deal to prevent accident on roads. In recent past, there was a great rise in the road accidents to the tune of 11.4 percent of the total vehicles on the Delhi roads, i.e. 11,50,000 vehicles on Delhi roads both light and heavy. This shows that road accidents are the biggest cause of the disability incidence after those who die in these accidents. In an over all assessment and assimilation of the information of this account they are generally the victims of head injuries and followed by complications, spinal injuries at various levels to the extent of quadriplegic, half body side paralysis, total amnesia, behavioral disorders and personality disorders.

It goes way back in 1982 when in thought of working on the lines of community education on the aspects of hazards of road accidents. I will not forget to mention that my institute authorities when I consulted to enrol myself as traffic warden with road safety cell of Delhi trafic police, did allow me take-up that study and make observations on that account to help reduce the handicaps on account of preventing road accident also my grateful thanks to the present director Sh R Prasad of the institute who time and again is always ready to allow me further the cause of the service to the handicapped in whichever way I have ventured to do, I may add that Sh R Prasad is the soul behind to encourage me to publish my first book on occupational therapy for physical injuries in 1979 and till today is giving me all opportunities and support to work for the cause of disability through occupational therapy at his institute.

Occupational therapists as designer: It is inherent in any occupational therapist after the study of the occupational therapy practice that one who is creative, innovative, perceptive to changes around become a useful and versatile occupational therapy.

As I have already said in the preceding paragraphs, that while educating road users on red lights on Delhi roads on hazards of road accidents and leading to various disabilities was not considered sufficient by me because while looking to the exposure of a pedestrian on road on Zebra crossings, it was just felt necessary that why should I not lessen this exposure pedestrian from vehicular traffic so that he is safe and reaches other end of the road safely. Immediately consulted the Deputy Commissioner Police Traffic on this and discussed in details the effects if we continued with the existing practice of Zebra crossing exposure to any pedestrian. It was agreed at length and I could succeed in blocking that exposure which helped to minimize the chances of the accident on that account. This was followed by re-routing the traffic flow accompanied by the haulting of all charted buses which also were threats to more accidents and hence disability on these roads of the area.

My emphasis is if there are no limits to act for any occupational therapy, the extent to which one can imagine is a concrete visible and the problems of the disability do not occur at all. In my opinion in our country, the disability is a permanent tax to one who suffers from it. So, therefore, the prevention and awareness are the answers for the future.

The suggestion made should be as far as possible an integral part of health care system in taking technology to doorsteps of the disabled persons.

APPENDIX 25: MENTALLY RETARDED AND SOCIETY

Integration of the mentally retarded into the main stream of life is utterly necessary to make them a part of society to which they owe a responsibility like any other normal human being.

Society is a group of families put together in a bigger context. Hence these approaches are to be made through the family members of the mentally retarded who must in first place, accept their disabled child so as to contribute their might in the direction, of the integration into the society, of their child.

As a result, the mentally retarded is made functionally, independent which can be looked after by occupational therapists as later is equipped with skills required to rehabilitate them into their main stream of life.

Mental retardation is a big chapter to cater to for anyone of us handling the rehabilitation science for this category of the disabled therefore, in this given limits of time some of the aspects relating to integration of these persons would be placed before.

Problems Outline as Viewed by Occupational Therapists

Occupational therapy with mentally handicapped is an approach quite different from that used in most other fields of disability.

For mentally retarded, the treatment objective is to develop latent potentialities and capabilities which never come to notice before and to provide them social education which enables them to take their place with confidence in unfamiliar surroundings.

In good old days, these retardates were employed on menial jobs where seniors supervised them with strict discipline imposed on them. Their idea was to keep them occupied all the while without leisure to make mischief. Perhaps it was because of poor concentration span of these persons. Since these retardates have hardly abilities to show/take inititive in jobs hence their obedience to do a particular task assigned is high.

The present day social system can no longer absorb such worker with limited intelligence in aforesaid manner and it is necessary to device a manner and system of training to fit them into employment, a way of social integration under modern conditions.

With all this in mind has given rise to the concept of:

- Day training centers
- Sheltered workshops
- Hostels.

For training the stable mentally retarded individuals to turn them into useful citizens and promoting integration into society.

Attitudes of Society

Retarded adult or a child has to live in a world of normal people around to live and work in close association with those people. All human relationships are two ways—A's attitude to B is in part determined by B's attitude to A—and the retarded person more than the non handicapped is sensitive to the manner in which the other people treat him at home, work and play. The life of the handicapped is made harder or easier by the attitudes of those around whom he moves and when community considers the making of provision for the handicapped out of community resources. The climate of public opinion determines whether that provision shall be generous or not.

Over all, we find that public opinion and feeling is against rather than for the handicapped.

Public attitude towards mentally retarded is very different. This category of the disabled is generally used for the purpose of the entertainment of the masses instead of a right projection of their image to society.

The mentally handicapped are tolerated or not in the light of highly irrelevant considerations. If they exhibit learnt social behavior and are readily accepted but if incompetent then institutionalizing is compulsory.

The worst social difficulty is that they are encountered by the mentally retarded whose parents are intelligent. He may be unacceptable in his class because cannot share his interests with others.

Factors responsible for the attitude can be understood in the following manner:

a. Amongst parents
b. Amongst Teachers at school
c. Amongst his peers around
d. Amongst his fellow workers at place of work
e. Amongst people around at home and public places.

Amongst parents: The attitude of the parents varies towards a retarded sibling than towards a normal one. The reason for this is that retarded may be a slow learner and may have delayed milestones during years of development. This may irritate the parents and they may not like and leave the child as they would have done otherwise. The child who is abnormal like this can appreciate this kind of ill feeling of his parents and may express rejection of their behavior by not executing their instructions.

Amongst teachers at school: The teacher has to work harder with retarded scholar in class than otherwise. This extra care, energy, attention requirement of a teacher is over demand as compared to a normal class. This is not generally taken in the spirit of the acceptance of a slow learner in the class which affects the teacher in her temperament towards this retardate.

Amongst peers around: The fellow children may not adjust with retardate as one of them. This way result into an attitude of discrimination and complete segregation of the retardate from their group. If it does not happen then the other children may tease him for his ill habits, poor concentration and poor pronunciation.

Amongst fellow workers at place of work: The place of work in general is considered a last place of journey coming to an end in rehabilitation of the mentally retarded. But to our surprise we do come across situations where the adult retardate is not accepted at all by office people. This lack of education to office people makes it imperative to understand the community. Education in mental retardation is yet too far from reaching them. Hence the problems of acceptance of attitudes towards mentally retarded.

Amongst people around at home and public places: The negative attitudes of family members and then of the public badly mares the measures to rehabilitate the mentally retarded. The positive approach is confronted by negative issue of feelings towards this category of the disabled.

The ill feelings of the parents mars the social acceptance of these disabled persons to such an extent that many children are so confined to four walls of their house that even the next door neighbor does not know that there is mentally retarded child in their vicinity.

I very strongly feel that the mass media—television and radio must be exploited to full along with a considerable involvement of press who also have social commitment to the society. It is now high time when such an action must be generated in its true sense to educate the society and community at large as to how mentally retarded can prove useful to the society after completion of the rehabilitation process of the disabled.

I fully agree to the statement that if learner has not learnt, the teacher has not taught.

The attitude of the professionals towards the mentally retarded should also go in conformity to the statement above.

The Informatory Management

To overcome above attitudes we need to have a multinuclear approach to the problem to enable each one of the society member to have a right type of temperament to understand and contribute towards fuller rehabilitation of the mentally retarded.

Institution Vs Community

While discussing this perhaps there is a silent challenge to integration of mentally retarded. I being an optimist will definitely like to advocate that institutional care is necessary to prepare the mentally retarded to face the community at large at some or other stage of the integration during rehabilitation planning. Hence the retarded must be trained for all possible types of eventualities he may come across in his life.

Management and care approaches: They may vary from case to case. However, for the purpose of understanding we may list as under:

  i. Prevent deterioration as far as possible.
 ii. Avoid habits harmful to themselves, to property or destruction.
iii. Assist in developing functional freedom.
 iv. Encourage purposeful activity and lessen dependence on others for personal help.
  v. Direct activities towards constructive channels if possible.
 vi. To achieve the above aims, the occupational therapist will:

  • Give their confidence and so attract their attention
  • Obtain their intertest so that they may imitate and cooperate
  • Stimulate purposeful and coordinated activity
  • Instruct in useful activities
  • Instruct in constructive activities.

The application of occupational therapy skills to achieve above and aims objectives of the treatment may also be marked by self-attitudes of the mentally retarded individuals as they have least realistic self-concepts. They even do not have on attitude about himself. Self-concept varies depending on the situation in which the mentally retarded child is. This also places them oddly in the society to learn confident living. The society is different opening for mentally retarded in different ways.

It is therefore, necessary that the social contact of the retardate may be more favorable after having come across different people around. There are sizable gains for retarded persons living in a society/community. The being of mentally retarded in a community affirms promise to keep more and more mentally retarded persons out of institutions and permit them to lead as normal a life as possible. Like any other normal individual the retarded also has equal rights of education, employment, voting and housing.

A normal life mans the right to enjoy the same privileges as any other citizen. These include obtaining licenses, insurance, recreation for example, on a nondiscriminatory bases.

Many unskilled and semi skilled jobs are available in the service area of hotels, hospitals and laundries. Bankers need helpers where these retarded can be employed who do not fall in the educable class.

Sheltered workshop can offer jobs which are paid work on industry sub contracts, such as assembling ball pens or toys and enjoy a sense of achievement. This economic satisfaction goes a long way in social rehabilitation of the mentally retarded. Employment of mentally retarded brings benefits to individual family and society.

Marriage of mentally retarded also is a social issue based on conceptions of society, whether they can be good parents? whether they can carry-out their relationship as wife and husband? which often perturb the parents of the mentally retarded who have a grown up child at home with problems on that account. They (parents) must immediately seek advice from the experts on this issue before the retarded puts them in any embarrassing situation on this account.

Due to poor mental competence, the retarded sometimes find themselves in criminal court where the parents and the professional will have to come forward to save the retarded from any unwanted punishment thereby saving their social image.

Like this, we see that mentally retarded is definitely a useful component of the society who is always keen to offer services to whatever way they are able to do. What needs today is the opportunity to the mentally retarded to show his worth and prove his worth and prove his abilities to society. It is therefore, my appeal to society at large that they should actively consider giving equal opportunities to this class of disabled also who owe a promise to come up to their expectation in productivity and national building like any normal person of this society.

APPENDIX 26: ASSISTIVE DEVICES

The assistive devices are given to all the handicapped individuals who find to carry-out their activities of daily living (ADL) with difficulty. The devices help them within their total percentage of the present inability. And, in some instances, these devices help a lot to make an unable patient an able one.

Indication and purpose: Often a patient is unable to manage an activity without special equipment or even to start without such aid. While every effort should be made to do without extra equipment, or at least to keep it to the minimum. It should be recognized that such devices, if wisely selected may increase speed and safety. It makes it possible to imitate an activity much earlier in the treatment program than will be feasible otherwise. Increasing activity earlier is also therapeutic.

Role of Occupational Therapist

When ADL treatment has advanced rapidly and has made great progress in use and acceptance, it is still a field in which participation is open to many interested persons. Not only doctors, occupational therapists, physiotherapists, nurses and patients themselves may become involved but orthotists and special technicians have been added to the team in many places. Interested volunteers and manufacturers have made many contributions. Today many designers and engineers are devoting their skills to help to solve the problems.

Occupational therapists today may participate on many levels with their skills in the house, tools and materials knowledge and understanding of various physical disabilities and physical function because they have the facilities of workshop available. Frequently, they may be called on to fabricate devices even if only temporary ones. Because of their interest in this field many occupational therapists have already made outstanding contributions today, because of the increasing supply of commercial devices. The gradual interest in the training of orthotists, the need for occupational therapist to make devices themselves is lessening gradually. However, in the role of evaluation of devices including testing and training the occupational therapist is and probably always will be key performer. Although he/she should continue to give assistance whenever needed, according to development in his locality or institution, the main emphasis of the role described here will be laid upon testing and training.

Psychological aspects: This aspect is of special importance and is of consideration of psychological reaction of the patient in relation to the use of mechanical aids or devices. Some of the factors found to influence their satisfactory acceptance and use are:

- i. *Interest:* May be influenced by any of the other reactions or by the patients feeling that he is sick and out do on duration and extent of the disability.
- ii. *Age:* May be a liability or an asset or may not be important.
- iii. *Reaction to the new and different:* Some persons are inspired by new ideas. The majority tends to favor accustomed and previously accepted methods of doing things.
- iv. *Cosmetic factors:* One of the goals of the rehabilitation is to give the greatest possible appearance of normalcy whenever it can be done.
- v. *Social cultural factors:* Feeling of the acceptance by the society at home or in some social gathering.

The Devices

Before prescribing any type of assistive device we have to keep many points in our mind which will lead to successful acceptance by the patient and purpose for which it is designed. The various points to be considered are:

Mechanical Aspects

The design or fabrication of a device may not be the responsibility of the occupational therapists. However, even if it is not, knowledge of essential factors enhances his own understanding of devices fabricated by others or of those available commercially. This does not mean that the occupational therapists should be expected to add all the skills of mechanical engineering to his own present training or that he uses only of his acquired bits of knowledge to infringe on the responsibilities of the other team members. It is suggested only that if he makes devices he should be equipped with as much know-how as possible.

If he participates only in testing and their method of fabrication is invaluable in getting expectation of performance of device itself and in knowing where to look for trouble spots.

Time: Patient's need varies time for the construction. If the patient's interest is ilicited try to supply the devices as quickly as possible. Waiting decreases his receptiveness. But beware of poor construction and unsuitable materials which reduce durability in case of operation. Breakdowns are frustrating also.

Materials: Select the material according to the patients needs. Weighing factors like weight, strength, flexibility, durability, washability, life expectancy and color against cost and method of fabrication and facilities for construction. Most of the new plastics and many metals can be handled successfully in a small workshop with a minimum amount of experience.

Construction: The key note is simplification and durability. The less complicated the construction, the more quickly and easily can one meet the demand. Durability results in fewer repairs and visits to the workshops. Both these needs are best answered through better knowledge of materials.

Operation: This factor of necessity go hand in hand with the construction. Usually simplication of construction means case of use. However, this may not be true in regard to sliding parts, where friction may have to be eliminated. And here we must refer again to the individual needs of the patients disability, intellectual functioning, manual dexterity and the environment.

Design: Depends upon all other factors plus the cosmetic needs. Good design has its foundation in the basic principles of good construction. Modern architecture offers many fine examples. Beauty of construction and function can go hand in hand.

Manufacturing Aspects

a. Extent and/or amount of use
b. Availability and cost of the materials
c. Interpretation of requirement of the devices for the production
d. Construction details
e. Operation or how to use it
f. Manufacturing goals
g. Estimate of potential market and distribution.

Training: Just as a person cannot be expected to drive a car properly without learning or to perform an acrobatic feast with excellence without repeated practice, so a person with a new device may need a period of training in its use. Never should a patient be discharged without the opportunity first to perform successfully whatever activity is undertaken. There are some cardinal rules:

- Learning something may take a long-time. It is a process, not an end result, so allow adequate time for practice
- Mistakes are a part of learning. If not repeated too often, they may even be helpful. They may remind us of precautions and may suggest that there may be better ways
- The patient may have valuable suggestions to offer. Listen to those carefully and objectively before rejecting ideas different from your own
- Keep alert to better and more effective methods of training. Enthusiasm properly controlled is always an essential
- Even though, careful planning has been given to designing a device in actual use, one may find that certain adjustments or modifications are necessity.

Therefore, it's the occupational therapist, who is the whole sole designer of these assistive devices which will solve all the problems involving disorganization of activities of daily living. They are the architects of the hopes of these disabled, a community of invalids.

APPENDIX 27: OCCUPATIONAL THERAPY FOR QUADRIPLEGIA AND PARAPLEGIA WITH SPECIAL REFERENCE TO SELF-HELP DEVICES

The rehabilitation process for spinal cord injuries is perhaps the longest for these patients who once get such injuries. There is more psychological stigma than actual awareness about the ordeal through which the disabled would have to pass through.

Such injuries are posing a constant challenge to the professional, involved in their rehabilitation because no single case of spinal injuries is alike. Each time, we face a quadri or a paraplegic means a new case as far as its needs and clinical picture are concerned.

These patients know some how that this is a long-term problem which has rendered them helpless and useless. Their morals is badly affected to the extent that they may completely turn uncooperative. If this happens, it is very difficult to keep them smiling with their life time disabilities.

The patients with paraparesis and quadri—paresis do not cause much anxiety even to the professionals but if those are plegias— perhaps each one of us knows well that it is a job indeed to make these patients smile and cheerful when knowing well that they have to live with their difficulties and problems.

Many of these patients develop associated problems which can be a serious hurdle to be crossed while being on the path of mangement. The complications like:

  i. Incontinence
 ii. Constipation
iii. Mobility problems
 iv. Ulcers
  v. Pressure sores
 vi. Lack of interest in life or no interest.

It is evident than when these couple with therapeutic management and care how tedious it must be for the handling therapist in occupational therapy which needs both physical and psychological participation in its activities. The activity being used as a treatment method while occupying these individuals on the activities which completely engross these patients that they get involved fully in the activity program and try to forget and broad over their inabilities.

When on bed in wards the patient activity program may be kept actively like—TV viewing on the films which show other such cases who came out successfully from distressful situations during getting disabled after spinal injuries. Narration of success stories of other such cases or photographs, etc. may be shown to them which keeps their moral up. A session of constant group or individual reassurance will go a long way in alleviating many of their problems by the occupational therapist. Why it is necessary is because the patient's psychological discomfort, might be a complete no cooperation from him.

I, as an OT have seen that most of the cooperation needed in cases of spinal injuries is much dependent on the former first rapport with the patient. We should not begin at once the therapeutic activity program. The first visit of injured to the occupational therapist would only limit to knowing each others interest in very informal manner. This may be give a way of at home session with the spinal injury patient. In this session, the two may talk for about 45 to 60 minutes for that day.

Next visit will be with a cheerful greet from the occupational therapist by addressing the patient by his/her first name. It helps break distance barrier and an intimation link is developed. Before that occupational therapist should get his/her on table for evaluation before actual treatment begins. It will be observed that it has done 50 percent of the total job when complete evaluation is done by the occupational therapist—thorough explain to the patient (in the language of the patient as far as possible) the details of the daily activities program in occupational therapy department. This not only makes the therapist know about his own planning for the case but patient gets to know properly what the program for him has been fixed up in that department daily.

Like this, the therapeutic sessions progress and continue for quite sometime when a time to think on the self-help adaptation or the adaptation to protect from injuries in both para and quadriplegics in case they have anesthetic feet adapted jean foot wear as explained also when the quadri or paraplegics are made to stand to improve their standing tolerance on account of anaesthetic feet the extra heel pressure involved in standing must get due attention with paded heels with side padded supports attached to padded band which encircles legs on both sides 2 inch above tendo-achilles. This will reduce to the minimum the cracking of heel skin or ulceration possibilities in these cases. These can be mass produced without difficulty as the materials are easily available in any equipped occupational therapy department of any hospital/center. The measurement depend from case to case The materials required are:

    i. Jean cloth 3" × 4" (in double layer)

    ii. Sponge/Foam 2.75" × 3.75"

    iii. Strip of jean cloth in size 1.5" × 8"

    iv. Jean cloth strip around leg 2" above ankles bent 1.5" × 9" with buckle on one side and eye lets on other end of the strip.

If can be washed with ordinary soap and water and can be ironed too if so desired.

This is adapted under garment to avoid ulceration on hips. The padding can be of foam which facilitate washing as well as drying very soon, if gets dirty. The material used is as under:

    i. Tericot/cotton cloth/spun in the size 20" × 20" in thee such pieces.

    ii. The foam sheet in the size 19.1/2" × 19.1/2" in one piece.

    iii. The elastic band 1" × 20" to the top of the under garments.

    iv. Velro or shirt press buttons (4 on each side) for making it easy to wear as hyper anesthesia and extra sensitivity cause difficulty to change these clothes in routine.

    v. These can be stiched in the department only by any occupational therapist after individual case measurement.

In case, where we need the catheter to be fixed accordingly opening has to be provided.

These types of under garments not only are comfortable at the hips but also provide extra care so as to eliminate chances of ulceration/redness due to inner easing pressure on these areas.

The changing of the clothes in these cases also is quite a bit of a job. It is generally seen that minimum two persons are required for changing clothes of the spinal injuries cases.

The design of their clothes especially for the quadriplegics may be like dangri with a difference that it may have shirt press buttons all around its edges right from top to bottom so that only one left and one right turn to the body of the quadriplegic may be given and one person alone cane change the clothes of the same patient.

The Material can be

   i. Tericot/spun/cotton, etc.

  ii. Shirt press buttons.

 iii. Thread and a sewing maching.

Assistance can be an adapted hand glove for the spastic hands especially when fingers cannot be extended by the patient voluntarily. This glove will help fingers keep extended at DIP and PIP joints. which will act as passive extension of these joints.

This glove will prove useful for these cases because they are not actively able to extend their fingers.

The material can be:

   i. Zean cloth (of the size of the hand of the individual with extension of the same piece up to lower one third of the fore arm).

  ii. Plywood/PVC (3 mm) of the shape of the hand above the PIP joints in both hands.

 iii. The piece of PVC or plywood at above will be inserted into the pouch provided to fit it snugly so that the glove when worn remain fit to keep fingers extended.

OT and Vocational Training Intervention in Spinal Injuries

It has been seen world over that spinal cord injuries form a big percentage of the various types of injuries come across by paramedical professional. The need to cater to one to one basis has been and is being felt in the present revolution of the total management care of spinal injured cases. There has been need for long for total rehabilitation care of such disabilities in this country. It is definitely a leap forward for the future and hope of the disabled person suffering from paraplegia and or quadriplegia. Till now, it was mere a hunt for the right type of professional to handle cases of spinal injuries in towns and cities of this nation. Some facilities for long term rehabilitation were existing with the development of such center, it will be a boon for spinal injuries cases.

The question now is how to develop services like occupational therapy, physiotherapy and vocational rehabilitation services for these disabled in future. If we consider one by one, we may view as under.

Occupational therapy/physiotherapy vocational training services: This will cover administrative management and rehabilitation of this disorders, which may be understood in the following perspective:

Administration

It should cover aspects of staffing, budgeting and equipment/ machinery and furniture requirement, etc.

1. *Staffing:* Physiotherapy/occupational therapy/VRO/UDC/ Assistant typist, etc. as the need may be.
2. *Budgeting:* Separate for physiotherapy, occupational therapy and vocational training in terms of salaries and all related for machinery/equipment, library, etc.
3. *Equipment/machinery:* Conventional may be combined with all latest computerized equipment in OT and PT and if any for vocational training (VT) also.
4. *Furniture:* There should be wood and steel mixed furniture with mica blends wherever possible in all attractive colors/shades. As far as possible, it may be rounded in shape to avoid any injuries in use of furniture during care, treatment, management and vocational training sessions. The size and other specifications will be on internal standards to unify this aspect also with care in any other part of the world.

Management Care

This may be understood on the lines: Acute, subacute and chronic stages which aims on the functional rehabilitation of such disorders.

1. *Acute stage:* Only up to the time, the patient is confined to bed aiming at proper positioning and support to the paralyzed parts of the body. When conscious then psychological handling to make him/her accept the fact that he/she has gone disabled temporarily or permanently after ascertaining his/her prognosis.

2. *Subacute stage:* During this stage, mobility is permitted in the case to came out of bed and go for toilet, go to department for treatment and also learn use of wheelchairs calipers and crutches, etc. as the case may be.

   In addition to above various activities of daily living (ADL) may be considered for purpose of training them with emphasis on functional independence in:
   • Bed activities
   • Wheelchair activities
   • Transfer activities
   • Ambulatory activities
   • Travelling activities.

   Maximum time needs to be devoted towards functional rehabilitation. In addition to above, the use of calipers and crutch training is also taken up which may be with slight knowledge on repairs of calipers for minor falls and crutches also so that the person does not need to waste time for minor—repair jobs to go to orthotics workshops including shoes repairs also.

3. *Chronic stage:* This stage reaches when these cases do not show much improvement or do not improve at all. There will be total acceptance of handicap by now which is coupled with a feeling to the vocationally independent in case they are not able to go back to their previous place of work or job. In such instances, there is need for the vocational counseler and of the vocational rehabilitation officer for these cases.

   It has to be taken into account that:
   • What is age/sex of the patient?
   • What is his educational background?
   • What is his/her socioeconomic status?
   • What adaptations/provisions need to be provided to such particular disabled person?

- What possible occupations, the patient wishes to chose to select on as means of livelihood. It may be well understood by us that as far as possible we must try to send him to job on which he was before if the disability permits. In my view success of rehabilitation on cases lies in hands of the disabled individuals to their previous occupations for which we might have to struggle as professionals.

This is also to consider that productive therapeutics and non productive therapeutics in occupational therapy management and care. Productive therapeutics will be that while therapy is being administered to the patient with the help of some useful craft activities, the end craft products of such cases should be sold on the sale counter of the department of occupational therapy to earn some money for the unit and more to give sense of accomplishment and utility to these case in the society. For this, the chronic stage cases can be picked up to make them economically independent themselves as far as possible. Another facet to this can be non productive therapy which only aims at remedial occupational therapy concern on muscle strengthening, increasing or maintaining range of motion (ROM) wherever possible in the affected parts of the body to release spacticity wherever present. It may also be taken care of that prevention of deformities are by provision of splints, calipers, etc. with surgical boots along with crutches or canes as the need be.

In upper extremity, the emphasis will be to keep all joints supple as far as possible so that muscles strengthening with therapy could be undertaken without much problem or no problem.

As upper extremity is mainly responsible for about 80 percent of our daily activities and functions, therefore, also needs more attention in its rehabilitation with or without self-help devices.

During off therapy session, there should be an active gymnasium, sports hall, recreational club and TV room for the recreation of these inmates and outdoor cases is also possible.

There may be concept of resident therapy team for these cases who do not have any body to look upon for their problems pertaining to the plans and need of each case. This is my own thinking on concept which I personally, feel that is viable if we so desire. Such a concept (whatever, amount of literature reference for such cases is done by me) does not exist at present in any part of the universe. We may like to consider it. This goes in addition to the day treatment hours in the center for selected cases where we feel we can achieve more faster and faster.

With this conceptual note I while concluding might add that rehabilitation of spinal injuries cases is such a dream which can come true if our intentions are clear.

Like this, we can do many more things to facilitate functional abilities. There can also be an effort put into device any to promote the abilities in self-care and self-help in spinal injury cases.

APPENDIX 28: ATTITUDINAL BARRIERS IN THE REHABILITATION OF THE PHYSICALLY HANDICAPPED (A PERSONAL VIEW OF AN OCCUPATIONAL THERAPIST)

An attitude can be defined as the intensity of positive or negative affect for or against a person, symbol, phrase, slogan or ideas. Thus, attitudes influence how a person behaves towards another person, thing or thought. If attitudes can be viewed socially as resulting in positive or negative behavior, then the occupational therapists, must be aware of one's own attitudes as well as those of the patients.

In fact, attitudes do influence the relationship between the occupational therapists and the patients. Since, the relationship is important for establishing a basis of intervention attitudes which are positively valued are desirable, whereas negatively valued attitudes are to be discouraged. The approaches are two way:

1. Attitudes in direct service
2. Attitudes in indirect service.

The direct service attitudes are:

a. Attitudes in evaluation: The attitudes affect the process of occupational therapy most directly. Therefore, attention focuses on intervention process beginning with evaluation. Attitude of objectively and emotional neutrality are the component of the evaluation without any personal feelings or values to interfere with reporting facts.

b. The evaluation phase offers an ideal time to establish an attitude of trust between the therapist and patients when therapist is sincere in her efforts, the patients is more likely to cooperate. The other attitude is the respect for other professionals contributions to the fact gathering process.

If, as above, the attitudes are not forthcoming they turn out to be serious barriers in evaluation, treatment, planning of the patients in occupational therapy department.

c. The various attitudes in terms of concern, right of determining his life goals, his weakness, right of the patients to privacy, patient confidentiality, protecting the patient safety, preventing further injury or illness, discouraging over dependency are which if not looked after carefully may cause barriers in program intervention. Attitudes in direct services are:

- Administration: The attitudes should facilitate administration and management of the program for the disabled in the department of occupational therapy.

- One important attitudes is respect for the patient as the focus of the concern failing which we may not get cooperation of the patient—a barrier in achieving progress further.

- To express concern for client care is expressed in the attitude that provides continous monitoring and assessment of the effectiveness of programs in occupational therapy. The concern is also expressed in the attitude that places a high value on continuing education of all staff members who are related to the rehabilitation of disabled, otherwise the barriers cannot be crossed at all or the professionals have to struggle to its maximum to achieve ones goals.

d. The supervisor must have an attitude that therapists/experts working together can provide a more comprehensive treatment program than can be provided by one person alone. If it is not kept so might prove a serious barrier in obtaining rehabilitative goals and objectives.

Also maintain respects for individual ideas and opinions to facility crossing any kinds of barriers if existing to prevent making of the program objectives.

The supervisor attitude, third in number is that values fairness and impartiality to enable evaluate the personnels on the basis of their duties and performance than on prejudices which might confront a barrier in the process of achieving goals.

The educator must adopt an attitude that respects the student as a professionals to be and support the growth of knowledge and skills involved in becoming a therapist any other discipline personnels if not so many be termed as a barrier in free learning situations of the professionals to be.

There are some of the attitudes of those supervising professionals to be and those who plan the program for the disabled but in addition to above, if we look into total dimension of the attitudes we find them in society, in vocational pursuits, in training places, in social gathering, public places, educational institution and where not.

- The additional barrier of the society toward the disabled is that they are not recognized in the true sense in the present times also. Say for an example: Nobody will accept willingly a disabled girl for matrimonial purposes. It is also sometimes a problem for disabled boys also but not very often.
- The attitudes are horrifying in vocational pursuits: The disabled professionals do not get much facilities in terms of adaptation of the various places/buildings, etc. wherever they are employed hence face also architectural barriers.
- The training places: Though might show reservations for such categories but are hardly welcomed unless by some or other kinds of pressures.

  The question of on the job training facilities also greatly face the acceptance barriers which do not allow the proper development in trade skills of the disabled. If not given full opportunity on this account shall seriously threat the rehabilitation program of the handicapped economically.
- The social gatherings many a times are places of insult, harassment, humilitations, etc. for the disabled persons owing to the lack of public awareness of such kinds which damages the courage and will of the disabled to live life like a normal person.

  Some of these individuals of the society will deliberately explore the happenings thus torturing the feelings of the concerned which might be a very painful segments to be narrated. Those who unknowingly do so are also damaging their courage to face the life/society before them with their defect/deformities and other handicaps.
- The attitudes are uncertain at public places, bus stops, shopping centers, cinema houses and clubs. As soon as disabled enters the field of vision of the individual causes a commotion in the vicinity and all eyes around turn to this disabled person with various

exclamatory signs which perturb him considerably. This may result into an attitude of totally withdrawn personality for future appearances at all above places thus hampering socialization of the disabled a great deal. This poses a big problem for the treating person in such instances.

• The educational institutions have hardly any positive attitudes for higher educational facilities wherever possible for the handicapped. The issues are evaded, wherever they can, on some or other pretext leading to a vaccum again in this area.

I very well remember the theme of one of the traffic police seminar in New Delhi on the education of citizens on traffic rules from early childhood as catch them young. I personally advocate the same idea that for effective cooperation and positive attitudes towards the handicapped, the integration of the disabled from very childhood is utterly necessary, except in cases where it is not possible at all depending the extent of the deformities and mental abilities. Therefore, every idea needs churning before it takes shape of a concept. A positive attitude to facilitate the barrier free rehabilitation of the physically handicapped is the utmost need of the house and call of the present times failing which we may place rehabilitation in tears.

APPENDIX 29: KEY NOTE ADDRESS

"He who calls me disabled is disabled himself" that is what I think about the handicapped.

1. I am indeed greatful to the organizers of this international conference to have given me an opportunity to address the learned participants in the fields of pollution, diseases and rehabilitation and also chair the session on rehabilitation.

2. I shall not hesitate to presume that such an august forum, rarely constituted must have discussed the multitude of problems relating to the rehabilitation of the afflicted due to pollution and diseases.

3. Pollution is very much responsible for causing of abnormalities, rendering the individual invalid either fully or partially, reducing his capacity to perform day-to-day activities. Thus, a situation arises where it is necessary to provide functional rehabilitation.

4. Diseases can be of various types causing variety of disabilitities functionally in a part or parts of a body, sometimes involving the whole of the body of the individual, which all of us are well aware.

5. In the case of instances, where pollution coupled with diseases affecting human body the results can be most damaging and nothing can be more drastic.

6. The total spectrum of disabilities brings into focus the need for rehabilitation planning. While thinking about rehabilitation planning, it is imperative to identify initially the areas of limitations a disabled individual is subjected to. The persons getting temporarily or permanently disabled have to meet various challenges in life to re-establish themselves, if not normaly but like normals.

7. We find a disabled person very uncomfortable and helpless in his situation of functional inability. Here we have to assess whether his disability can be arrested or maintained from deteriorating and how his mobility can be ensured. This is a physical and medical problem. The other strains on his personality arise from his psychological stress for adjustment in society and also his financial dependence on society. Here we confront with socioeconomic problems.

An expert in the field of rehabilitation has, therefore, to tackle a multitude of problems covering diverse fields.

8. Therefore, when we think of rehabilitation we face an uphill task for, the disabled of various physical disability groups the deaf, the dumb, the blind, the orthopedically handicapped, the mentally retarded and the spastics. The extent of possibilities of rehabilitation varies from group to group. In some cases, it can be confined only to physiomedical problems while in many cases, the problems are physiomedical and socioeconomic.

9. In this situation, I confine the modus of rehabilitation to a few specific programs:
   a. Measure to arrest further deterioration.
   b. Measures to maintain the existing functional abilities.
   c. Measures to create functional abilities where they do not exist with the help of various kinds of the devices/aids.
   d. The integration of the individual in the society at the earliest so as to minimize any complexes affecting his personality.
   e. Securing economic freedom.

Program drawn keeps these as objectives I believe will go a long way in the total rehabilitation of the disabled.

Rehabilitation

As is well known, rehabilitation refers to an adaptation process following injury or a disorder and habilitation refers to a learning process for persons born with a disability or having one very early in life.

Rehabilitation process is a goal oriented and individualized sermon of services designed to assist handicapped individuals to achieve vocational adjustment—A care point of many psychological reactions developing in disability cases.

Aspects

Individualized process: Every person is unique, psychological and personal reactions to disability, therefore, vary from individual to individual. Similarly, no two persons have exactly the same needs or potential each having unique assets, ways of coping with goals. Hence, rehabilitation is an individualized process.

To make rehabilitation, an individualized process required integrating a myriad of specialities and resources into a comprehensive approach for serving the whole individual. It is generally accomplished in two ways:

One way is the team work and approach among professionals which depends on a client's needs, coordinating the specialized skills of the various team members involved in this process.

The second way is by using a generalist known as a rehabilitation councilor who not only provides services but also coordinates multidisciplinary services on behalf of the individuals. This councilor must be aware of everything going on and must direct the rehabilitation process into the master plan.

Service or goal oriented process: It is also known as servantial service delivery for, it emphasizes the delivery of services at proper time and in most appropriate servance for each person. Servance generally envisage evaluation, treatment, training, job placement and post employment services.

Interdisciplinary nature: Since rehabilitation deals with the whole person because professions are specialized and composed of categories rehabilitation is necessary interdisciplinary in nature.

Socioeconomic implications: Depend on value and dignity of the individual human being for participation in the privileges and responsibilities of the respective citizens offer immeasurable justification for public rehabilitation program. Rehabilitation can lead to self-respect, to improve personal, family and social adjustments and to the elimination of despair, frustration, bitterness and grief. It can provide meaning for one's life in addition to relief from financial stresses or the humiliation of being unable to carry on an acceptable social role.

There is further need to develop more social awareness regarding disability and the disabled so as to have proper feedback of the existing services. There has to be growing need always to better plan the program for the handicapped which should help them to attain their respectable social status. Their social acceptance hastens the total rehabilitation process enabling the handicapped to accept himself as a part of the remaining society. The rehabilitation resources must be built-up to cope-up with the growing demands of these services wherever possible.

Rehabilitation services: Since, the disability is either a physical or mental condition which limits a person's activities or functioning, it requires early attention so as to minimize obstacles to maximum functioning. Rehabilitation services aim at removing or reducing the handicapping conditions resulting from disability rather than the disability itself.

The eligibility criteria for rehabilitation services is:

- Existence of physical or mental disability conditions which constitute or result in a substantial handicap to employment
- Reasonable possibility that rehabilitation will benefit the individual in terms of employability.

It is further stated that the handicap must relate to employment and must be linked to the disability. While considering employment of the disabled it is emphasized that any laws governing employment must be amended from time to time so as to quicken the process of vocational rehabilitation.

- I have, during my career as a professional felt that the rehabilitation services suffer implementation.

There has to be bridging of the gap from hopelessness to usefulness of these individuals and contributing to national building. The attitudinal behavior towards the disabled should be positive.

A lower limb amputee is refsued all those jobs which he can do with his hands—to the job requirement his disability is not a handicap so where is the handicap. But only the attitude which does not permit this disabled seek reasonable employment. Most of such instances mount the growing anxieties of the disabled further and force the later to either commit suicide or develop purely a negative approach to total rehabilitation planning.

- *Short courses for placement and home management*: I strongly feel here that for proper implementation of the services so human as rehabilitation, the personnels from each rank and file must undergo refresher courses/orientation courses which must expose the experts or others related to the process to the growing needs of the disabled persons so as to understand individual case on its individual merits.

  So I feel about the courses for the parents/relatives/patients themselves which should impart information on various kinds of services available for them in their country and home management of the disabled in order to enable them to really view and recognize their roles in the successful rehabilitation program planning of their children/relatives.

- *Society and rehabilitation*: In the concept of total rehabilitation of the disabled society has a prominent place. Society being the cradle of development of personalities it should have a proper orientation to assist, help and guide the disabled to function as a normal human being.

- *Importance of publicity media*: In order to achieve that society plays a comprehensive role in the total rehabilitation planning of the handicapped and the media services are to be exploited to its maximum. The media as you all know has the maximum range to cover most of the total population which otherwise is not possible but might be very very expensive proposition to think.

The media—TV, radio and newspapers have a social commitment to which they have not been exploited to the full so far. I personally feel, why it should be difficult to film the process of rehabilitation sciences and show if not daily at least on alternative days the kind of services and treatment modalities which are available for different kinds of the disabilities of the handicapped in the particular region of the country.

It is strongly felt that all such platforms where rehabilitation of the handicapped is discussed in context of the social awareness of the masses, the media services must be utilized in projecting the same to the society by way of showing the films relating to treatment process of the handicapped individuals, etc.

It is indeed true that the services which are available in ones country remain unknown due to lack of publicity through media. In addition, each region must have one principle information center to disseminate information to those who are interested to know about facilities available for the rehabilitation of the disabled.

In conclusion of this address, I humbly appeal to media that they have a concern and social commitment to the cause of the handicapped and generation of an awareness in the minds of people of the possibilities and advantages of rehabilitation of the disabled and different kinds of the services available in the country for the rehabilitation of the disabled who are our brethren.

Index